Missing Management

Also by the author, available from Amazon in both paperback and Kindle versions

Riddles in Accountable Healthcare: A Primer to Develop Analytic Intuition for Medical Homes and Population Health

and

How to Ask and Answer Questions Using Electronic Medical Record Data

Missing Management

HEALTHCARE ANALYTIC DISCOVERY IN A LEARNING HEALTH SYSTEM

Eran Bellin

ISBN: 9781074850029

To my students who have become my teachers.
"Much have I learned from my teachers,
More from my colleagues,
But from my students, most of all."
—*BABYLONIAN TALMUD, TAANIT 7A*

Table of Contents

"A system in which science, informatics, incentives, and culture are aligned for continuous improvement and innovation, with best practices seamlessly embedded in the care process, patients and families as active participants in all elements, and new knowledge is captured as an integral by-product of the care experience."[1]

Introduction

The learning health system (LHS) is composed of three concepts—system, health, and learning.

System

A system is a construct both recognized by those who work within it as well as observable by those nonparticipants who wish to study it. The association of the word "learning" with the word "system" implies a conscious entity that organizes material and personnel assets to deliver specific services to achieve defined outcomes. The coordination of people and services requires a clear statement of specific goals, a measurement of process delivery, and an outcome. While it might be argued that some part of systemness could emerge from the proper manipulation of economic incentives, with reliance on an "invisible hand," precluding the need for a central authority, complex engineering, and adaptive coordination requires human intervention.

Gross incentives can focus attention and provide the means, but some consciousness must decide on the priorities, supervise, assess, and iteratively implement.

Unsupervised providers and health care agents acting in their own financial interest have the perverse incentive to discover inhomogeneities in law and practice to maximize profit and, as a by-product, frustrate emergent social good.

Health

The second concept is health. There is a spectrum of goals here, and it is critical to limit scope or else be distracted by our good intentions. Health care classically provides immediate relief of an acute clinical need, such as an acute fracture of an arm or the onset of cancer or a heart attack. Health care is composed of those processes that attempt to alleviate pain and reverse the condition if possible (and if not possible, to attenuate its impact).

Health care has a preventive component as well. A health care system engages with a patient early in his life when there is no evidence of target organ damage, but there is evidence of a remediable risk factor such as high blood pressure or high cholesterol that, if remediated, could preclude or significantly delay the onset of clinical disease.

Preventive health care can be expanded to include advising patients on high-risk behavior, such as smoking cessation and obesity reduction, with the hope that the advice will result in behavior change.

It has been recognized that social determinants of health, such as housing or food insecurity, can be drivers of health care delivery costs. The homeless might seek food and shelter in the emergency room, especially in wintertime. The poor asthmatic might find summer heat intolerable, requiring air conditioning in order to stay out of the hospital.

Efforts to ameliorate those social determinants as a cost intervention strategy can become part of the considerations of a health system trying to maintain cost control. Pushed to the ultimate extreme, employment can be thought of as the ultimate source of health, providing income, meaning of life, and social stability for the individual and family. The danger of pushing the definition to this extent is that by including all human need within the rubric of health care, those activities that are uniquely under the engineering control of the health care system are ignored in favor of glitzy aspirational social determinants.

Health care systems have a predilection for taking on boutique, high-PR-value social projects that distract from the more prosaic areas for which they have clear and exclusive responsibility. The core operations continue inefficiently, failing to provide value, while the institution distracts the public—and itself—from its failure to deliver on its core zone of responsibility. I will focus on health care delivery and demand systemness of this delivery.

Learning

In this book, we will work through examples of the sort of questions a learning health system could ask, examine how to turn the question into a formal query, and provide a first order analysis. The provided analyses are not complete by design. I will point out the biases, weaknesses, and potential next analytic steps. I will also point out how the next step might not be analyzing available data but rather obtaining new data with sufficient specificity and potential for generating meaningful action.

It is important not only to know how to pose the question but to have the software that lets those most proximal to the patient clinical experience—those who should pose the question—be able to do so and not be held hostage to the inertia of special data access privilege (priesthood of data access[2,3]), arcanum of SQL, or privilege of institutional rank to demand attention.

As you begin to empower curious, ethical, and committed actors in your learning health system, you will rapidly find deficiencies in programs and in the management of the activities necessary to achieve goals you might want to set—deficiencies ignored by the usual regulatory processes. This can be frustrating and, in the wrong system, punishable. The mediocre system lives in a Panglossian "best of all possible worlds," with highly intelligent and well-defended players who support the status quo and are unaware of their collusion. Breaking the delusion of perfection, or even of adequacy, does not immediately endear you to them as there is no immediate return to the bottom line. Choices must be made, and disagreements among the well-meaning are inevitable. The title Missing Management is chosen to highlight the natural consequence of this exploration and the need for leadership that has the vision and courage to tolerate the discovery of their own inadequacy and the cognitive dissonance that precedes redemption.

We do not claim to have instantiated the complete vision of the learning health system, but after 15 years of advanced informatics support (Clinical Looking Glass[3,4]) and collegial efforts in PDSA cycles, we are in a position to imagine what such a system would look like and how it would use information. The chimeras of an easy solution with electronic medical record (EMR) purchase, or registry building, or the implementation of the fad of the moment for best outcomes, is giving way to careful observations at the gemba, methodical analysis, and iterative interventions with evaluation. We are not at Nirvana, but in the words of Churchill, "Now this is not the end. It is not even the beginning of the end. But it is, perhaps, the end of the beginning."

Our Fractured World

No longer do we have the mythical doctor with continuity over time and continuity across acute episodes. We parse patient relationship into inpatient, outpatient, and intensive care, as well as acute procedural intervention. I have seen on YouTube an abomination[5]—an end-of-life conversation with a robot, the human image with a stethoscope appearing in an imbedded robot monitor, the patient lying in the intensive care unit. No history together at all. No human shared experience. No human touch. The ultimate compartmentalization. This is truly something no patient wants, but we have been sliding into Gomorrah for years. The care of the individual is lost in myriad silos with no animating global vision or purpose, just short-term, nonlongitudinal goals. Financial reimbursement reinforces this perversion, favoring the acute, intensive, and short-lived while implicitly encouraging purposeful ignorance of anything that might complicate acknowledgement of the short silo's task completion. In such a world, feedback is narrowly constrained, and opportunities for learning and improvement to cross siloed goals are lost. Emotional coherence providing for the patient's spiritual and emotional support is now no longer a responsibility of a long-term relationship but a task checked off on someone's work list—a horror that has lost any semblance of humanity.

The learning health system must learn not just how to detect disease, reduce cost, and provide preventive care. It must also learn how to provide care—human care—a challenge all the greater for the prevalent perverse incentives. It seems that we are seeing a clinical community with members increasingly on the spectrum. Their MCAT scores are rising. Their curriculum vitae are becoming fancifully more impressive. But lost in all this is an understanding of what it is to care and to be responsible. This value is not being nurtured in medical schools that are morphing into unapologetic trade schools accelerating completion in three years rather than four by robbing the college years of the flexibility for broader experience. It is not clear that we had the solutions in the past, but it is clear that we are not attending to them now.

Eran Bellin, MD
eranbellin@gmail.com

Surveillance for Intervention and
Learning for Diabetes, Hypertension, and
Hypercholesterolemia: The Chronic Trackable
Triad of Population Health

Diabetes

A population of diabetics must be followed for at least two years to evaluate management success. I will work through a specific example of incident diabetics in a large collection of primary care clinics to demonstrate how one might effect meaningful evaluation to support a learning process for follow-up intervention.

I create a group of incident diabetic patients in 2016 who are under care of one of 24 Montefiore Medical Group (MMG) outpatient clinics.

Using Clinical Looking Glass,[3,4,6,7] I apply the following case definition for incident diabetic patients in the Montefiore Medical Group. I provide the number of unique patients as the additional criteria are added.

1. Patient with MMG outpatient visit in 2016 (N=152,894)
2. Patient with a HgbA1c≥6.5 within 0–6 hours of the outpatient visit (N=20,927)
3. Patient without evidence of diabetes diagnosis 1–3,650 days prior to the diabetes defining HgbA1c (N=4,150)

Gestational diabetes is not included in the diabetes diagnosis set. The first time the patient achieves these criteria is the index date.

The screen shot from Clinical Looking Glass is provided in Figure 1.

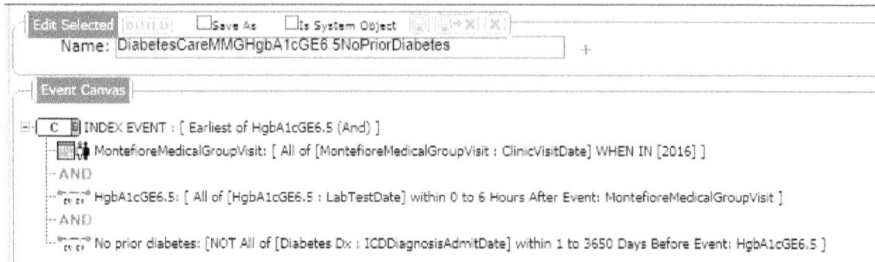

Figure 1. Clinical Looking Glass criteria for incident diabetics, 2016 MMG group

A histogram of new onset diabetes defining HgbA1c is provided in Figure 2.

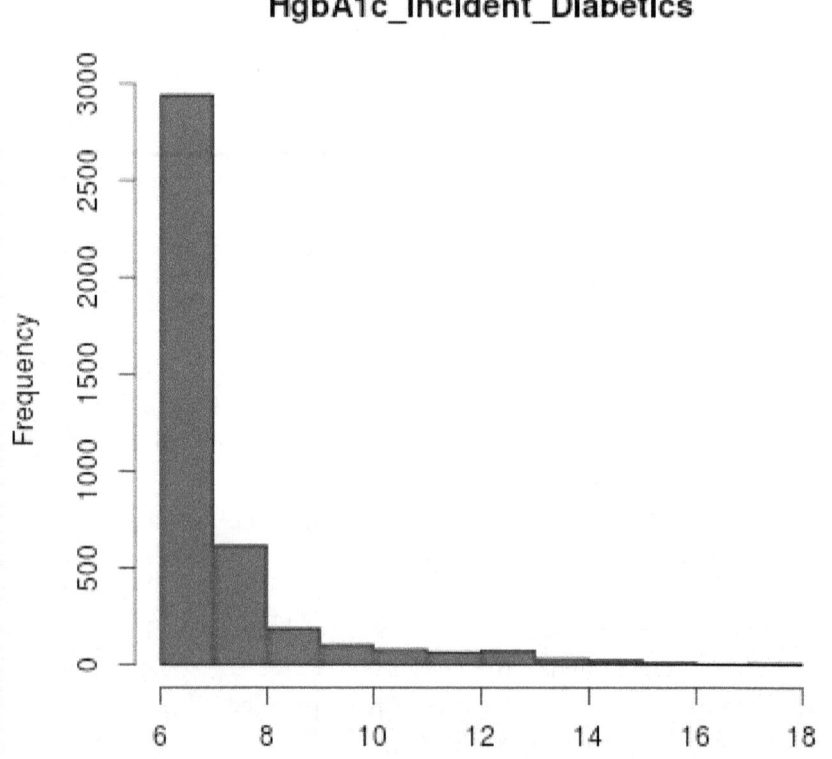

Figure 2. Histogram of incident diabetes defining HgbA1c

Table 1. Frequency of HgbA1c ranges for new onset diabetics

HgbA1c Incident Diabetics	Count	Percent
*[6.5–7.5)	3,350	80.72
[7.5–8.5)	318	7.66
[8.5–9.5)	131	3.16
[9.5–10.5)	78	1.88
[10.5 or greater)	273	6.58

*[includes the value in the range;) excludes the value in the range

For each cohort member (Figure 3), collect all the HgbA1c values in the interval 365–730 days after the initial HgbA1c (Figure 4), and then identify the minimum and the maximum HgbA1c experienced in the time window (Figure 5).

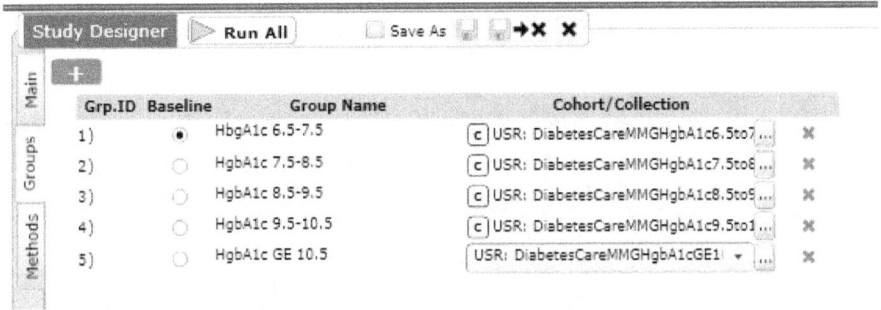

Figure 3. CLG Study Designer enrolled cohorts

Create an analysis definition that looks for *all* HgbA1c 365–730 days after the first.

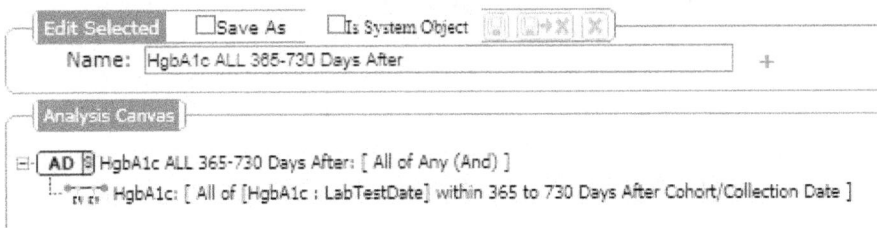

Figure 4. Analysis definition finds all HgbA1c in time window 365–730 days

Figure 5. Select the minimum and maximum value from the interval

Then build two tables. The first table shows in the rows the patient count in initial HgbA1c ranges, and the columns show the minimum HgbA1c in the 365 days to 730 days after the index.

Table 2. Patient count by initial HgbA1c ranges and minimum repeat ranges 365–730 days after initial HgbA1c

	Minimum HgbA1c Ranges 365–730 After Initial								
Count of Initial HgbA1c	[0–5)	[5–6.5)	[6.5–7.5)	[7.5–8.5)	[8.5–9.5)	[9.5–10.5)	[10.5–20)	Missing	Grand Total
[6.5–7.5)	6	1826	317	36	20	6	14	1138	3363
[7.5–8.5)	1	72	81	25	14	3	6	127	329
[8.5–9.5)		18	27	17	10	8	6	52	138
[9.5–10.5)		11	15	11	7	5	1	28	78
[10.5 or greater)		37	26	32	20	16	26	117	274
Grand Total	7	1964	467	121	71	38	53	1462	4183

Table 2 is an optimistic view of success. The best HgbA1c 365–730 days after the first is used to characterize the patient. Of the 78 patients initially in the 9.5 to 10.5 range, 5 remain in the 9.5 to 10.5 range. This display allows you to identify the number of patients who have not improved enough and pull out their names so you can target them for intervention. In addition, the existence of 28 missing patients is deeply disturbing as they have not been retested in the one to two years post their diabetes incidence.

This table is a useful tool for those organizations that are serious about population health. Rather than focus on the provider as the source of the failure, this patient-focused map provides the signal to the health system that can focus appropriate nonphysician resources to assure timely follow-up—social worker, diabetes educators, and engagement specialists. The erroneous default assumption by many is that the target of the intervention should be the physician for whom a signal either as a message in his inbox or a penalty in his salary should somehow stimulate him to fix this issue. This is foolish, especially when the relevant resources that need to be brought to bear are either nonexistent or not under his control.

A less optimistic view of clinical success is provided in Table 3 as it looks at the worst HgbA1c in the 365- to 730-day window. For those initially in the 9.5–10.5 range, instead of five remaining in that range in our optimistic Table 2, we now see six.

Table 3. Patient counts by initial HgbA1c and maximum repeat ranges 365–730 days after initial HgbA1c

	Maximum HgbA1c day 365–730 After Initial								
Count of Initial HgbA1c	[0–5)	[5–6.5)	[6.5–7.5)	[7.5–8.5)	[8.5–9.5)	[9.5–10.5)	[10.5–20)	Missing	Grand Total
[6.5–7.5)	3	1679	400	61	32	14	36	1138	3363
[7.5–8.5)	1	47	76	31	17	11	19	127	329
[8.5–9.5)		10	24	10	14	16	12	52	138
[9.5–10.5)		8	8	14	8	6	6	28	78
[10.5 or greater)		26	22	19	20	21	49	117	274
Grand Total	4	1770	530	136	91	68	122	1462	4183

Frankly, using either table twinned with a defined targeted intervention would be an improvement for most health systems aspiring to learning health system status. It is at this table level, visible and sensed by the system itself, that targeted interventions can be planned, implemented, and evaluated.

As an example, the health care system might decide to put into place a remediation plan for those who have failed or gone missing. Using the most optimistic view to reduce false positives and waste of remediation outreach services, the learning and managing health system might identify the patients identified in highlighted cells Table 4 as worthy of effort.

Table 4. System view identifying remediation targets (highlighted)

Count of Initial HgbA1c	Minimum HgbA1c Ranges 365-730 After Initial								
	[0 to 5)	[5 to 6.5)	[6.5 to 7.5)	[7.5 to 8.5)	[8.5 to 9.5)	[9.5 to 10.5)	[10.5 to 20)	Missing	Grand Total
[6.5-7.5)	6	1826	317	36	20	6	14	1138	3363
[7.5-8.5)	1	72	81	25	14	3	6	127	329
[8.5-9.5)		18	27	17	10	8	6	52	138
[9.5-10.5)		11	15	11	7	5	1	28	78
[10.5 or greater)		37	26	32	20	16	26	117	274
Grand Total	7	1964	467	121	71	38	53	1462	4183

These are the patients who are still greater than 8.5 after two years of interaction or are missing follow-up after initially being greater than or equal to 8.5. This system action view identifies people for system outreach with novel methods potentially independent of the action of their primary care provider.

In Table 4, 14+3+6+10+8+6+52+7+5+1+28+20+16+26+117=319 people out of the initial 4,183 (7.6%) require *system-*, not *practitioner-based*, salvage intervention. If instead you allow the practitioners to have the first shot at improvement, you can build a scaled down (i.e., less costly) intervention targeting a smaller group for remediation. Of course, the system can also work to make the practitioners more effective in their first efforts, but this informatics remediation action view now clearly demarcates the system salvage mission from the initial efforts.

This tabular style is of use even when you are looking only at the present population at the present time when you are trying to determine what ought to be done

Table 5. Patient counts by initial HgbA1c and BMI ranges

Count of Initial HgbA1c	BMI of Incident Diabetic					
	[0–25)	[25–30)	[30–35)	[35–40)	[40–60)	[60–120)
[6.5–7.5)	248	841	893	549	461	25
[7.5–8.5)	26	77	88	52	47	5
[8.5–9.5)	8	41	34	13	23	1
[9.5–10.5)	6	22	17	16	8	0
[10.5 or greater)	29	73	58	44	30	0
Grand Total	317	1054	1090	574	5691	31

with two variables of concern, say HgbA1c and BMI. Use the cut points for BMI of less than or equal to 25, 30, 35, and greater than or less than 40.

From Table 5, decide who might require bariatric surgery intervention or who might be benefitted by directed exercise.

It is now understood that one might be appropriately less aggressive in HgbA1c control for the elderly, so looking at the population by age range (Table 6) is useful to determine who might be better left alone.

Table 6. Patient counts by initial HgbA1c and age ranges

	Age of Incident Diabetic			
Count of Initial HgbA1c	**[0–40)**	**[40–60)**	**[60–70)**	**[70–120)**
[6.5–7.5)	323	1,635	840	565
[7.5–8.5)	26	96	46	23
[8.5–9.5)	36	138	66	36
[9.5–10.5)	15	35	21	7
[10.5 or greater)	45	156	49	24
Grand Total	445	2,061	1,022	655

You might forgive the 70-year-olds with HgbA1c of 6.5 to 7.5. Benign neglect might be the appropriate approach as we are taught in medical school, *primum no nocere (first do no harm)*.

Hypertension

Introduction

Hypertension is recognized as a major risk factor for stroke and cardiovascular disease[8-11] with its control a justification for preventive medical care visits. Assessing and monitoring hypertension control using the patients' EMR footprint requires case definitions and metrics that tolerate imperfect reality, shine a clear light on the deficiencies, and are resilient to support surveillance with the advent of better BP measurement technologies and protocols.

To effect preventive medicine population hypertension control by twinning EMR information with a health care delivery system's action arm infrastructure requires a clear notion of objectives and their measures.

A good group of metrics should provide three capabilities:

1. Identify patient populations for whom interventions are required.
2. Rapidly detect the effectiveness of new interventions.
3. Properly characterize maintenance of success.

Using clinical data from a large number of urban medical clinics from a single health system, I evaluate longitudinal hypertension control success as I imagine will be required of future stewards of health care.

Methods
Study Population

Montefiore Medical Center, the University Hospital for the Albert Einstein College of Medicine, has 20 internal medicine and family medicine clinics providing primary care in Bronx, NY. Eleven (55%) are federally qualified health centers (FQHCs).

A single Epic EMR system supports inpatient and outpatient care with all data flowing into Clinical Looking Glass,[3,4,7] a user-friendly advanced temporal cohort builder application supporting on-the-fly creation of cohorts and longitudinal outcome analyses. Reusable temporal analytic patterns allow for the rapid assessment of dichotomous and continuous outcome measures.[3,4] All analyses were performed in the restricted mode as a limited data set under the Health Insurance Portability and Accountability Act of 1996 (HIPAA), in accordance with Institutional Review Board (IRB)-reviewed protocol 2014–3985 EMR as medical textbook, Albert Einstein College of Medicine.

Each patient's address is geocoded to census block with neighborhood socioeconomic status (SES) calculated using the method of Roux.[12] The neighborhood SES variable is presented as the number of standard deviations distant from the mean SES of New York State census blocks.

The race/ethnicity self-designation variable is provided as the percent of the population with ethnicity (dichotomized as Hispanic/not Hispanic) and given priority over race.

Blood Pressure Assessment

Systolic blood pressures recorded within six hours of an outpatient visit were identified as outpatient blood pressures and were the only ones considered in this study. We were interested in assessing longitudinal outpatient care and did not want to include blood pressures associated with hospitalizations or emergency department visits.

The definition of "hypertension" was purposely chosen not to reward those clinics with poor follow-up rates. Some surveillance definitions require two blood pressures measured at different outpatient visits before declaring a patient hypertensive. That criterion rewards those institutions that fail to provide adequate follow-up, forgiving them their first and only hypertension reading. I also avoided any criteria requiring multiple blood pressures with some rule[13] (average of three, last two of three, at rest, specified arm) as once again these requirements make it impossible to initiate a surveillance process for health care systems that have not yet refined their process.

By choosing an available simple measure, single systolic blood pressure,[14] I am able to profile every clinic. Of course in the first year, post blood pressure measurement protocol refinement such as multiple blood pressures per session,[13] automated office-based measurement,[15] or home-based ambulatory measurement,[8,16-21] I would expect to see remarkable improvements. However, once improved, the new standard will provide a stable measure of control and comparability. Our objective is to build a detection system that will reward systems to actively evolve protocols for surveillance, detection, and intervention. Transient increase in the initial detection of hypertension in a population with a subsequent unearned exaggerated sense of success in year two is of little concern if, by tolerating such reporting delusions, we ultimately create a meaningful surveillance system with reproducible and comparable results in years three and four.

Analysis

I divided the patient population seen in 2016 into established or new patients based upon whether or not they were seen at least once between 5/5/15 and 12/31/15 and into middle-age or elderly cohorts for ages 40–60 and ≥60, respectively. The first systolic outpatient blood pressure in 2016 was considered baseline. Final blood pressure was the last outpatient blood pressure recorded 1–365 days after the first.

Using JNC 8,[22] the target systolic blood pressure for those middle age (40–60) is <140 and for the elderly (age≥60), <150. Thus, age-dependent hypertension is defined as a single blood pressure in middle age of ≥140 and ≥150 in the elderly.[22]

I demonstrate our approach using the new patient population. By focusing our analysis on new, rather than established, patients, I avoid the problem of overweighting the study population with failures[23] due to resistant hypertension, a consequence of biologic, emotional, or social causes. The hypertensives in new patients are those expected to achieve the greatest proportion of hypertension control success with the clear implication that failure in this group testifies to a serious primary failure of accountable care.[4] While the responsibility of the failure may legitimately be shared between the patient and the health care system, it is the health care system that must consider the steps for process failure remediation. In addition, the number of incident hypertensives discovered in 2016 constitutes a useful number when planning future demand management in this population.

Importantly, new patients have not been functionally "trained" by the health system with bad habits reciprocally developed and reinforced by patients and their providers. New patients can develop new rules of engagement with new protocols and new expectations, preventing trained hopelessness and mutually reinforced health care behavioral incompetence.

Patient description is provided for all patients in these clinics (both established and new) and in a separate column for those who were new (Table 7).

Table 7. Patient description—all patients and new

	All Patients	New Patients with BP in 2016
Clinics Federally Qualified Health Center	N=20 N=11 (50%)	
Population	N= 101,732	N= 31,082

Age
    40–60
    ≥ 60
	
	54,172 (53%)
	47,560 (47%)
		
		20,393 (66%)
		10,689 (34%)

Age Percentiles:	(5th, 25th, 50th, 75th, 95th) (42, 50, 58, 68, 82)	(5th, 25th, 50th, 75th, 95th) (41, 47, 54, 63, 78)
Females	65,832 (65%)	18,235 (58.7%)

Race/Ethnicity
  Black
  Hispanic
  Other
  Unknown
  White
	
	36,176 (36%)
	35,756 (35%)
	10,093 (10%)
	9,960 (10%)
	9,747 (10%)
		
		10,416 (34%)
		10,153 (33%)
		3,619 (12%)
		3,769 (12%)
		3,152 (10%)

Language
(Primary)
  English
  Spanish
  Other
  Unknown
	
	80,136 (79%)
	18,704 (18%)
	2,190 (2%)
	702 (1%)
		
		24,772 (80%)
		5,211 (17%)
		804 (3%)
		295 (1%)

Neighborhood Socioeconomic Status (# of standard deviations from NYS mean)	Percentile (5th, 10th, 25th, 50th, 75th, 90th, 95th) -8, -7, -6, -2, -1, 0, 1	Percentile (5th, 10th, 25th, 50th, 75th, 90th, 95th) -8, -7, -5, -2, -1, 1, 1

BMI	Count	Cumulative Count	Cumulative%	Count	Cumulative Count	Cumulative %
>40	8,213	8,213	8.2%	2,337	2,337	7.5%
35-40	11,858	20,071	20%	3,260	5,597	18.4%
30-35 (Obese)	25,844	45,915	45.8%	7,718	13,315	43.8%
25-30	34,986	80,901	80.6%	10,857	24,172	79.5%
(Overweight) <25	19,437	100,338	100 %	6,228	30,400	100 %
Missing	1,394			682		

Results

Final Blood Pressure Metric

In this first metric, we focus on new patients who are hypertensive in their first blood pressure measure. We then follow each person for a year of follow-up and record his last blood pressure in the interval. Longitudinal failure is defined by either failing to have any blood pressure measured in the ensuing 365 days or by having a last blood pressure in the interval above the age-appropriate threshold. This last blood pressure is determinative of hypertension control. It is a longitudinal failure because once a patient is identified as needing intervention, the one year of follow-up provides adequate time for interventional success.

Of 20,390 middle-age patients, 4,444 (22%) were hypertensive. Of the hypertensives, in 1,365 (31%) patients, final blood pressure continued to demonstrate hypertension, and 1,186 (27%) patients failed to have any repeat blood pressure. A total of 58% failed to demonstrate longitudinal hypertension control.

Of 10,689 elderly patients, 2,674 (25%) patients were initially hypertensive. Of the hypertensives, 762 (29%) had final blood pressure that continued to demonstrate hypertension, and 579 (22%) failed to have any repeat blood pressure. A total of 51% failed to demonstrate longitudinal hypertension control.

Health care delivery systems are challenged to decide on priorities for follow-up. Until now, our use of a single systolic blood pressure value of ≥ 140 in middle-age patients weighted all patients equally and explicitly imposed our actionable threshold notion on the reader. To obviate this, I create a matrix of middle-age longitudinal failures (Table 8) with initial blood pressure as row names and final blood pressure as column names. I provide in each cell the number of longitudinal failure patients requiring follow-up meeting row-specified initial blood pressure cutoffs and then either lost to follow-up or meeting the column-specified final blood pressure. I provide both the number of patients requiring follow-up and, in a select number of cells, the percentage of the row-defined hypertensives. The matrix allows those charged with making resource-allocation decisions the ability to properly prioritize targeted intervention expenditures.

Table 8. Longitudinal middle-age failure matrix counts including missing (N=4,444 hypertensive new patients)

		Last Systolic BP within one year of first 2016 BP					
		Missing	*≥200*	*≥180*	*≥160*	*≥150*	*≥140*
First	*≥200*	10	12	19	26	36	40
Systolic	*≥180*	43	45	65	100	138	172
Blood	*≥160*	267	274	308	457	618	784
Pressure	*≥150*	577	584	630	861	1,145	1,478
2016	*≥140*	1,186	1,194	1,248	1,545	1,965	2,551(57%)

The middle-age longitudinal failure matrix demonstrates 457 patients with an initial BP≥160 and either a missing subsequent blood pressure or a final BP≥160. A similar matrix for the elderly (Table 9) demonstrates 627 patients.

Table 9. Longitudinal elderly failure matrix counts including missing (N=2,674 hypertensive new patients)

		Last Systolic BP within one year of first 2016 BP				
		Missing	*≥200*	*≥180*	*≥160*	*≥150*
First	*≥200*	14	17	23	35	46
Systolic	*≥180*	68	71	111	186	239
Blood	*≥160*	312	317	389	627	807
Pressure	*≥150*	578	584	674	1,028	1,340 (50%)
2016						

Acute Control Metric

To evaluate an intervention's success to control hypertension in the hypertensive middle-age patients, I perform a time-to-outcome analysis with a target of first systolic blood pressure <140. This calculates the cumulative percent of patients who have achieved the target outcome by a defined elapsed time (30, 60, 90, 365 days). This cumulative-incidence calculation is the complement of the Kaplan-Meier statistic,[24] allowing the analysis to remove from the denominator those who are censored by death or administrative censorship while still extracting available information before censorship.

While administrative censorship only becomes a concern when patient populations are assigned to specific organizations for management, as functionally occurs now in managed care organizations, the time-to-outcome metric is robust and ready for the day when patients are assigned and then reassigned. Until reassignment, hypertension control is the responsibility of the original organization.

We demonstrate this cumulative incidence of hypertension control in those initially hypertensive in Table 10. Because the cohort is well defined and follow-up performance is determined quickly (at 30, 60, and 90 days), the health care delivery system can rapidly evaluate a new intervention's initial effectiveness.

Table 10. Elapsed days from initial hypertensive BP measure until first age-appropriate BP target

Elapsed Days	Age 40–60, Target<140, N=4,444	Age≥60, Target<150, N=2,674
30	14%	20%
60	24%	31%
90	30%	38%
180	42%	52%
270	49%	59%
365	54%	64%

The astute reader may have noticed in Table 10 in middle-aged hypertensives a 365-day success rate of 54%, which is greater than 42%, the complement of the failure rate of 58% calculated in the final blood pressure method above.

Why the discrepancy?

This discrepancy is the result of the fact that the first metric considers only the last value in the interval of 1–365 days to define success, while the time-to-outcome analysis seeks the first evidence of success independent of any final result. When early success is achieved but not sustained by the end of the follow-up interval, the two metrics diverge.

In the middle-age cohort, 2,412 (54%) at some point achieved blood pressure control but 487 (20%) lost that control by the time of the final measure. 1,893 (65%) retained control, and 32 (1.3%) had no follow-up BP after initial success.

When there is a repeat blood pressure after the initial success, I provide the number of elapsed days between the first evidence of hypertension control and final systolic measure (Table 11) for those who lost control and those with persistent control.

Table 11. Number of elapsed days between first evidence of BP control and final BP (age 40–60)

	Loss-of-Control group	Preserved Control Group
<1 day	18 (3.5%)	873 (45.4%)
1-30 days	27 (5.2%)	62 (3.2%)
≥30 days	442 (85.1%)	1,891 (49.7%)

Of interest, I found 1.5%, 2.2%, 2.4%, and 3.0% of the patients with a success within 1, 6, 24, and 96 hours, respectively, after the first measurement. This suggests that had the physicians recorded multiple blood pressures in the first BP ascertainment, the diagnosis of hypertension might have been avoided.

In elderly patients (2,674) with baseline hypertension, 1,698 (64%) at some point achieved hypertension control, but 342 (20%) lost control by the time of the final measure. 1,333 (79%) had persistent control with 23 (1.3%) having no measure after the initial success. The number of elapsed days between the first evidence of BP control and final BP is provided in Table 12 for those who lost control and those with persistent control.

Table 12. Number of elapsed days between first evidence of BP control and final BP (age≥60)

	Loss of control group	Preserved Control Group
<1 day	3 (.9%)	434 (34.7%)
1–30 days	19 (5.8%)	36 (2.9%)
≥30 days	305 (93.3%)	780 (62.4%)

Maintenance Metric

Blood pressure control sustainability is critical as the clinical impact of hypertension is affected by chronicity over years. A different metric is needed to evaluate the quality of blood pressure control maintenance that will summarize all the blood pressures fairly across an interval without artificially giving primacy to the final or first blood pressure.

Time in range[3] (TIR) is a method in Looking Glass that evaluates each individual's blood pressure trajectory by drawing an interpolated line between recorded outpatient BP values, when those values are close enough to permit interpolation, and carry forward the last value for a user-defined period when the last value is not close enough to interpolate. This allows us to infer a daily blood pressure or a missing value. Using user-defined and named ranges of blood pressure, the analysis sums the days experienced in each category (see Projection to x-time axis [Figure 6]) and then uses those sums to calculate the percent of time spent in each category. A sensitivity analysis can be performed by altering the user-defined intervals.

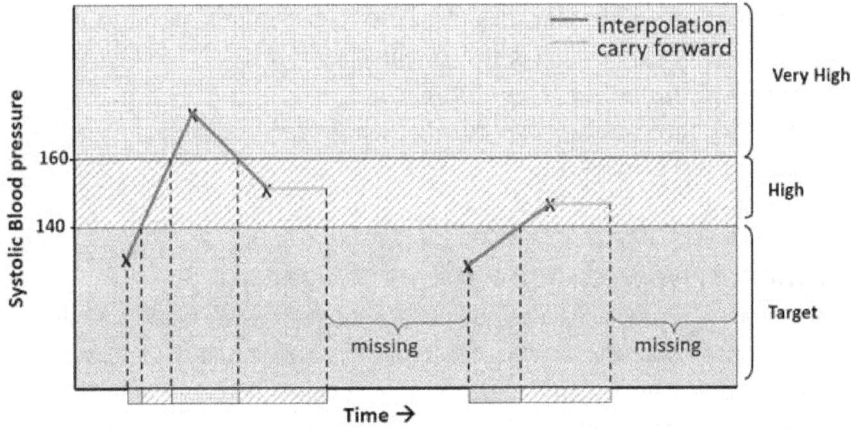

Figure 6. Time in Range method accumulates time in user-defined blood pressure categories

Adequacy of control is defined as the percent of time the cohort maintained its blood pressure in the ranges of interest. As an example, we have chosen 365 days as the interval for both interpolation and carry forward and demonstrate the result of Time in Range analysis (middle age Table 13, elderly Table 14). In middle-age hypertensives, BP was in the acceptable range only 37% of the time. Bootstrapping[25] the original data 5,000 times reveals a 95% confidence interval of (36.1%, 38.4%). 12% of the time, the cohort BP was in the 160–180 range.

Table 13. Percent time in BP range for middle-age patients initially hypertensive followed for 365 days

BP range	0–140	140–160	160–180	180–200	≥200
% of Time	37%	48%	12%	2%	0.4%

Table 14. Percent time in BP range for elderly patients initially hypertensive followed for 365 days

BP range	0–150	150–160	160–180	180–200	≥200
% of Time	45%	25%	24%	5%	0.9%

We can also use the TIR analysis to focus on the experience of patients individually. If we ask which patients maintained control for 66% of the year (i.e., were in control for 8 months of the year, thus giving each patient four months to bring their hypertension under sustainable control), we find that only 34% (1,512/4,414) of the patients achieved control for at least 8 months.

In elderly patients, 41% (1,098/2,674) of the patients had control for at least 8 months of the year of follow-up.

Additional Hypertension Patients of Concern

In addition to longitudinal failures, additional hypertensives are found among those initially normotensive who develop new onset hypertension in the follow-up year. 982 (6%) of 15,944 initially normotensive in the middle-age cohort and 627 (8%) of 8,014 initially normotensive in elderly became hypertensive. There were 9,876 and 5,755 repeat blood pressures available on the normotensive cohorts, respectively.

Established Patients

While our focus has been on hypertensive new patients, established patients had startling longitudinal failure rates: 48% (3198/6570) failures in middle age and 42% (2,929/7,032) failures in the elderly. However, the cause of the failure was different. New patients were more likely to suffer failure due to loss to follow-up, rather than to measured BP failures with proportions 45% (1,764/3,891) and 24% (1,489/6,127), respectively and an Odds Ratio of 2.6 (95% confidence interval 2.4, 2.8).

Discussion

The large number of longitudinal failures and new onset hypertensives among those initially normotensive suggest that a serious effort is necessary if we are to realize the population health benefits of hypertension control. The current model of scheduling patients for outpatient follow-up visits, rather than aggressive telephonic outreach with home blood pressure monitoring, seems to be failing.

Limitations

There is considerable variability in any single blood pressure measure with home measures often recording lower pressures.[26] This, however, does not minimize the implication of either untreated hypertension or inadequately assessed clinic-based blood pressures in patients with a higher likelihood of hypertension. The medical literature of the last decade, some of which is referenced in the bibliography, is filled with metaphoric hand-wringing on lost opportunity,[9,10,27] but surveillance reporting using the metrics we have described is not the norm.

The time-in-range measure makes the assumption that the actual blood pressure changes in a straight line between measures, which is, of course, untrue. But in the words of the great statistician Box, "All models are wrong, some are useful."[28] So it does give us a first-order notion of interval control. TIR does have a defect. It is very sensitive to blood pressure results that are far apart in time. In a situation where the patient has two office visits separated by many months, with the first visit having only one blood pressure recorded and the second with three blood pressures recorded within minutes of each other, it is the first blood pressure of the three that will drive most of the time-in-range calculation.

To remediate this weakness in the future, when multiple blood pressures are the rule, the clinician will have to decide upon a single representative blood pressure (average, best of three, etc.) for each clinic visit so as to allow the time in range to calculate its blood pressure range occupancy properly.

Conclusion

Value-based purchasing in health care is relatively easy when you are dealing with an episode of care—say, the elective hip replacement that bundles the replacement joint itself, hospital and rehabilitation session, medication, and physical therapy. Many technical deliverables are subject to this quantum-of-care and quantum-of-cost model with the market and payers driving down price. But these are situations where the intervention and outcome are relatively short term, with historically huge waste and inefficiency all completely under the control of the health care delivery system.

By contrast, in chronic disease management, the challenge is long term and dependent upon the whims of an often-unwilling patient who does not experience motivating short-term consequences, such as those found in a painful hip. Financial and health benefits are delayed consequences beyond the short-term financial interests of health care delivery systems or their governmental payers. This is what preventive medicine failure looks like hiding in the shadow of extraordinary medical technology, surgical miracles, and triumph over infection and some cancers. Its remediation awaits thoughtful surveillance and an action arm providing a home ambulatory measurement, scheduled escalating telephonic interventions—a consequence of clear institutional accountability with targeted funding.

Elevated Cholesterol: Medication Persistence

n the chapters on diabetes and hypertension surveillance, the reader was shown how to track the important values of characteristic laboratory tests and findings. In this chapter, I consider the question of how to track adherence to treatment. I assume that the patient has been initially properly determined to be in need of cholesterol control through medication, and I assume that once determined, this need is lifelong. The next step is to determine adherence to therapy so that the learning health care system might target those who are not adherent for additional engagement. The sort of engagement—email, phone call, group classes, or a physician reminder to reach out to the patient during an office visit—will be determined by the learning system in an iterative evaluation of cost effectiveness, the priority of which will be determined in the budgetary context of other potential interventions.

Of course, the most straightforward manner to determine adherence is to obtain from the pharmacies or pharmacy benefit plans the fact of prescription fulfilment. How many times a year, with how many pills, was the patient dispensed the medication of interest (in our case, the statins)? Most health care systems do not yet have this fact available to them.

In the interim, using EMR data with prescription, we can at least determine who has not returned to the physician for at least one prescription in the years 1–2 after the initially documented prescription, thus identifying those at high likelihood of nonadherence. More complex modeling, which I have done, can address this issue by counting the number of pills prescribed, refills, and duration to create a longitudinal view of percent of year covered by daily pill availability, but I will use a simpler method to identify egregious outliers certainly requiring our attention.

In this exercise, I will focus on patients with hypertension in 24 primary care medical groups who were prescribed statin agents within 180 days after their recorded elevated blood pressure.

The case definition as before uses a singleton systolic blood pressure as determinative.

1. Individuals aged 40–59 who have a systolic blood pressure greater than or equal to 140—middle-age hypertensives.
2. Individuals aged 60 or above who have a systolic blood pressure greater than or equal to 150—elderly hypertensives

The blood pressure must be recorded within six hours of an outpatient office visit to make sure that we are looking at outpatient blood pressures and not inpatient or emergency room measures.

11,728 middle-age and 10,966 elderly hypertensives were identified.

We will now assess whether a patient was prescribed a statin within 0–180 days after their high blood pressure.

To create the groups of statin medications, we will use the Explore function of the CLG software and use the FDB pharmacy hierarchy (Figure 7).

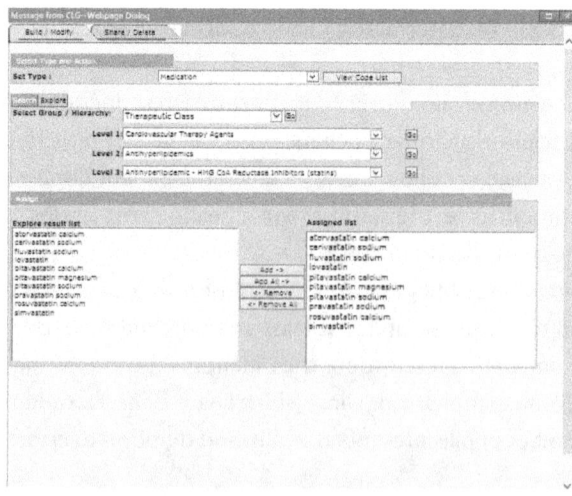

Figure 7. Identification of statins using FDB hierarchy

I save the set and add a new condition line to each cohort that looks for the presence of a statin prescription within 0–180 days of the blood pressure finding (Figure 8).

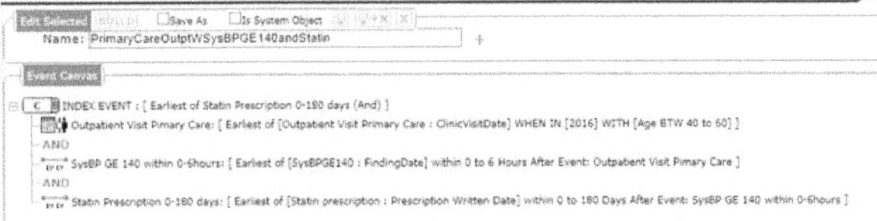

Figure 8. Middle-age hypertensive cohort MMG primary care sites with statin prescription

2,894 middle-age and 5,004 elderly hypertensive prescribed statins in the year 2016 are identified.

Now find the percentage of those who are still on medication in the interval of 365–730 days after the index prescription.

Bring the cohorts into the study designer, and follow those patients for 730 days for the presence of an outpatient prescription for a statin. However, require a blackout period of 365 days so that you will not recognize any statin prescribed in the first year—only a statin prescribed in the second year (Figure 9).

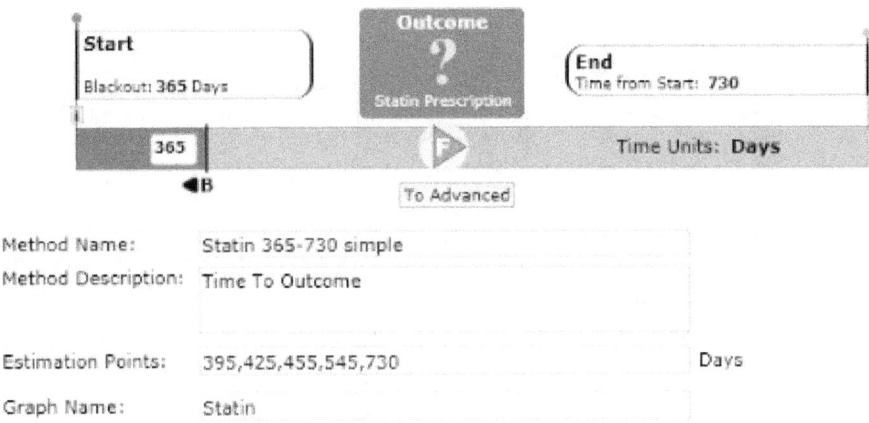

Figure 9. Time to Statin prescription over 730 days with blackout period in first 365 days

The resulting Time to Outcome graph and table reveal that by the end of the second year, 76% of the middle-age and 79.2% of the elderly hypertensives are still being prescribed a statin at least once. The elderly seem more adherent (p=.013), but importantly, even with this most forgiving of adherence metrics (you need only one prescription annually to be considered adherent), 21–24% of the population is not adherent to statin therapy (Figure 10).

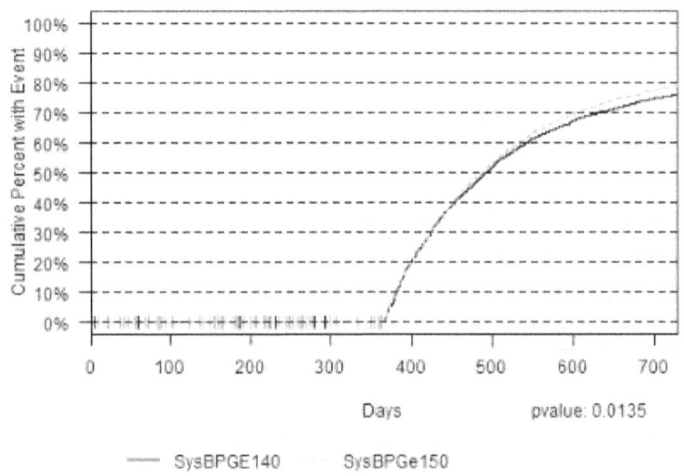

Cummulative % with Event	395 Days	425 Days	455 Days	545 Days	730 Days
SysBPGE140 (baseline)	18.3%	30.3%	41.1%	60.6%	76.0%
	(16.9,19.7)	(28.6,32.0)	(39.2,42.8)	(58.7,62.3)	(74.3,77.5)
SysBPGe150	17.7%	30.1%	41.3%	62.5%	79.2%
	(16.6,18.7)	(28.8,31.4)	(39.9,42.6)	(61.1,63.8)	(78.0,80.3)

Figure 10. Time to outcome for outpatient statin prescription days 365–765 after index statin

An entity committed to population health might view this finding as indicating a need for patient engagement and for seeking real-time prescription fulfilment data, so a more sensitive and timely metric could be used to track and respond to non-adherence.

LHS: What Do You Want to Know? What Are You Prepared to Do?

n the first three chapters, we reviewed population metrics for diabetes, hypertension, and elevated cholesterol, the three horsemen of the apocalypse of early cardiovascular mortality and stroke.

By creating meaningful metrics of control within a time frame providing ample opportunity, the LHS is in a position to determine which subgroups should be targets of public health preventive medicine efforts. One might want to concentrate on those patients who started at very high levels of abnormality and after adequate elapsed time did not achieve even a modicum of control. Consider those with HgbA1c greater than or equal to 8.5 who still were at 8.5 or above in the two-year follow-up period or were lost to follow-up. One could select patients aged 40–65 to achieve the best long-term benefit. One could identify obese diabetics—those with BMI greater than or equal to 35—and target them for specific diet, exercise, and ultimately surgical intervention. Similar approaches could be obtained for hypertension and elevated cholesterol.

Who should create and then look at these metrics? Who should be responsible, and what should they be responsible for doing?

The usual approach of dashboards and their public attribution of failure to the primary care practitioner, while in some sense is emotionally satisfying, is probably misguided as a sole approach. The physician in his—at best—15-minute interaction two to four times a year does not have the contact time or the ability to engage aggressively and consistently with the patient. How is the physician supposed to bring the patient back to the office for an office blood pressure check? Should the physician harangue his patient? This would not be too clever. Should the physician develop a patient-centered alliance on a single issue during the short clinic visit when there are many other issues to address? While this is the correct answer to multiple-choice exams for continuing medical education, studies have shown, unsurprisingly, that as the number of clinical issues with preventive medicine import rise, the likelihood of achieving guidelines goals in all of them tends to drop.[29] Clinical inertia is the expected outcome of reliance upon the standard office visit approach.[30]

Another approach would be for the responsibility for first surfacing the failure and then addressing it to reside with the learning health system (LHS). Let the LHS identify its own failures and recognize the physician as an asset to be properly managed, rather than as a whipping boy[31] to accept the blame for the sins of the delivery system and its nonadherent patients. Let the LHS find the solutions.

Perhaps this would include, in the case of hypertension, assigning the failing patient to a nurse- or physician-centered telephonic home blood pressure follow-up system. The patient would be engaged in a rapid, personal, quality improvement cycle where the patient takes ownership of his condition with daily blood pressure measurement and weekly blood pressure reviews with a nurse or doctor. Together, the nurse or doctor and the patient could, in algorithmic scripted interactions, overcome clinical and personal inertia. This is a formal referral to a process of weekly monitoring of daily collected blood pressures, weekly scheduled review of those blood pressures with a health advocate, and rapid escalation of medication every two weeks (or as appropriate determined by drug half-life) under the control of a clear algorithm with televisits with the physician. The clinic might cycle its own primary care physicians as the telehealth physician every third month to familiarize him with the algorithms and to encourage properly escalating care for those patients not yet in telephonic support so that the number of patients who need this remediation intervention would be reduced.

This intervention is part of the long-term reeducation of the physician and patient on how chronic clinical conditions are first brought under control and then maintained through ongoing personal surveillance at home, first intensively and then at longer intervals. It builds a different model of detection, intervention, and maintenance—quite alien to the present-day, physician-office, visit-centric approach.

To make these interactions time efficient, there would have to be a way for the appointments to be set up through a smartphone application and scheduled after usual patient work hours. Physician work hours could be more flexible to provide night coverage and staggered work hours.

Once control is achieved, the patient could be required to enter his results in the application, which would maintain automatic surveillance until a steady state is achieved.

A comprehensive process would include planning for medication delivery to the home so that the escalation of medication is not dependent upon the patient's willingness to go to a pharmacy and pick up his meds. We can imagine next-day delivery by Amazon Prime.

Once stabilized the medication will be delivered at 90-day intervals. Hypertension, diabetes, and cholesterol could have intensification and maintenance models that would be intrinsic to the learning health system.

But note, this is not about the LHS undertaking a randomized controlled trial or learning some grant-funded eternal truth shared through academic journals. It is about the LHS recognizing human frailties—of both patient and physician as well as local cultural realities and using technology and logistics (next-day med delivery) to overcome these weaknesses. The LHS must monitor its own performance over time and note when the intensification or maintenance is failing.

It must begin to see its physicians as fallible assets embedded in a complex and unsupportive environment and must change that environment to make this fallible asset successful. It must also be able to ultimately identify the recalcitrant patient who is unable to be remediated and then make difficult decisions that include the possibility of writing them off forever or for some time-out period rather than continue to expend resources (see next chapter). This latter possibility will be a necessary outcome with proper documentation as systems take real responsibility for achieving outcomes and must come to the realization that some people cannot be saved from themselves.

By having an explicit list of failures and the justification of the Do Not Save list, the LHS can, at intervals, make specific, targeted outreach to this group as well to see if new strategies might be successful.

Who Will Pay?

The notion that the LHS will address, through risk-factor reduction, preventable cardiovascular disease, the benefits of which are only visible on a decade's horizon, requires a mandate and dollars. Health systems make their money by expensive and profitable tertiary and quaternary care. Bundling the opportunity for these health care systems to access their lucrative source of revenue by requiring that they capture the population in financial, capitated arrangement is a strategy into which we are slowly evolving. The problem, however, is that the evolution is slow, and there is no guarantee of risk-factor remediation unless it is an explicit deliverable demanded in capitated systems. Indeed, requiring risk-factor remediation with surveillance and interventions would basically end the fee-for-service solo practitioner who could not provide this deliverable alone—although you could imagine a short referral for a three-month intensive intervention to a company specializing in such interventions.

To what extent such mandatory engineering is acceptable in our political system is yet to be explored. We could imagine even in a fee-for-service system that companies would arise that could provide the short-term intensification care and short-term surveillance that would then be explicitly paid for only for successful outcome by the payers. The patient would be offered an opportunity to leave their primary care MD for a short interval to undergo "clinical optimization boot camp" and be returned to their usual care, or they would be offered an alternative system of care once they have achieved their goal.

I suspect that a patient given the opportunity for an intensive intervention by a system that demonstrates focused care supported by integrated-care cellphone applications might never go back to the old style of physician office-only intervention.

The kick-start to this approach must come from funding the episode of intensification and paying only for success. The idea of true pay-for-performance—that is, not paying if the patient does not get better—has old roots[32] and should be considered.

Mammography Screening Outreach: An Early LHS Failure and Its Implications

Modification of an Unpublished Contemporaneous Report by Stephen Kulovits and Eran Bellin

n 2003, more than a decade and a half ago, the following effort was undertaken to improve breast cancer screening using mammography. While it was far less successful than hoped, it raises important philosophic questions as to the responsibility of an LHS.

This is an abbreviated and modified report by Stephen Kulovits and this author, reproduced with permission. This author takes responsibility for the abridgement.

Breast cancer screening has been shown to reduce breast cancer mortality.

The purpose of this effort was to systematically improve mammography screening rates of women in our network. We reviewed our administrative database to identify patients eligible for mammography but for whom, by claims data analysis, we were unable to find evidence to indicate that mammography had been performed. We used a standardized escalation protocol of telephone calls in an attempt to contact these women and schedule mammogram appointments at their convenience.

Background

Montefiore Medical Center, the University Hospital of the Albert Einstein College of Medicine, located in Bronx County, NY, is an academic medical center and integrated delivery system. It is composed of 3 hospitals, discharges 70,000 patients, and provides over 2 million ambulatory visits annually.

The Montefiore Integrated Provider Association (MIPA) is a legal entity that engages in full-risk contracts with area health plans. CMO, The Care Management Company, LLC, is a management services organization that oversees the administration of these contracts for the MIPA. In 2003, over 100,000 MIPA members had their care managed by CMO under these full-risk arrangements. A member is defined as someone who has selected health insurance through a payer contracting with the MIPA, has a benefit plan that is included in that contract, and has selected a primary care physician who participates in the MIPA.

Methods

This study was approved by the Montefiore IPA Quality Improvement Committee, which is part of the governing structure of the MIPA.

Definitions

Eligible Member: A member was defined as eligible for contact if they were female between the age of 48 and 69 who was a member of MIPA and had been continuously enrolled for 6 months prior to selection and for whom no record existed in our claims payment system of having a mammography in the past two years. This record would have been in the form of a processed claim or encounter. An individual was still eligible if they had had a single gap in enrollment not exceeding 45 days.

Contacted Member: A member was defined as contacted if the interviewer was able to speak with the eligible member on the telephone. Interviewers used scripted questions to determine eligibility for a mammography appointment.

Contacted/Mammography Eligible: A member was defined as contacted and eligible for mammography if the member was successfully contacted and confirmed that she had not had a mammogram in the last two years. They then attempted to schedule an appointment. The outcome of that scripted conversation then led to a member being placed in one of three categories:

- No appointment made—offer of appointment not accepted: The member refused our offer to make an appointment.

- No appointment made—member claims to have an appointment already scheduled: The member claimed to have a future mammography appointment scheduled within 3 months from time of telephone contact and refused to make an earlier appointment.
- Appointment made: Interviewer successfully made a mammography appointment for the member.

Contacted/Mammography Ineligible: A member was defined as contacted and ineligible for mammography if the member was successfully contacted and confirmed that they had had a mammography in the last two years. While we are aware of the concept of *telescoping*, where the actual date of the mammography is further in the past than the member recalls,[33,34] we elected from a practical perspective to accept the member's information. We did attempt to determine dates and locations of reported mammograms.

Not-Contacted Member: A member was defined as not contacted when after 6 telephone call attempts, using the telephonic protocol, the interviewer failed to speak to the member.

Reasons for failure to contact a member were logged as follows:

- No answer: Telephone was not answered within 10 rings.
- Answering machine: Telephone call was answered by an automatic voice system.
- Member not available to speak: Telephone call was answered by someone other than the member, and the member was not available to come to the phone.
- Disconnected: Interviewer heard a recorded message that the number they dialed had been disconnected or was no longer in service.
- Wrong number: Telephone call was answered by someone who informed the interviewer that the person they were seeking was not at that number.

Study Sample

A total of 6,153 members were determined from claims data as eligible for mammography.

Selection of sample to survey
A random sample of 505 names was drawn from the study sample. Each of five interviewers was then provided a listing of 101 members for telephonic outreach using the standard protocol.

Selection of Imaging Center
Collaborating with our imaging center, we were able to schedule appointments immediately while on the phone with the member at a day and time convenient to the member. Appointments could be made as early as the following day.

Selection of the Interviewers
Five customer service liaisons were selected from our call center to perform the telephonic outreach. All were employees of CMO, currently providing both inbound and outbound telephonic customer service. All were women, as we felt that a member would be more comfortable discussing their mammography history and accept an appointment for a mammography from a woman. One of the five interviewers had herself undergone mammography.

Training of Interviewers
To ensure that the interviewers were well versed on the benefits of mammography and early-detection strategies, training meetings were conducted, and relevant materials were distributed and discussed. Interviewers were provided a tour of the imaging center to familiarize them with the waiting area and dressing and exam rooms, as well as to meet with the front desk staff, technicians, and physicians. As a result, the interviewers were able to describe to the members what they might expect to experience.

Telephone Call Protocol
To maximize the numbers of women reached by phone, we created a telephone contact protocol of escalated assertiveness. This involved attempting to contact each member 6 times. Following any unsuccessful attempt, the caller would try a day and time that was assumed to offer a better chance of finding the member home. At the

completion of the call protocol, the member would either be defined as contacted or not contacted.

Table 15. Telephone escalation routine

Telephonic outreach protocol	Day of Week	Time of Day
1st attempt	Weekday	Between 9am–12pm
2nd attempt	Weekday	Between 12pm–6pm
3rd attempt	Weekday	Between 7pm–9pm
4th attempt	Weekday	Between 7pm–9pm
5th attempt	Saturday	Between 10am–2pm
6th attempt	Sunday	Between 7pm–9pm

Protocol for Incorrect or Missing Telephone Numbers

If no number was available in our system for a member or the number was found to be incorrect (e.g., wrong number, disconnected), the caller then attempted to search in the medical center's clinical information system and local telephone directory for an alternative number. If no other number was found, the member was defined as not contacted.

Conversation with Member

When speaking with the member, the interviewers followed a script designed to accomplish the following:

- Confirm the member's identity
- Confirm the member's eligibility for mammography
- Provide information regarding the benefits of mammography
- Facilitate appointment scheduling with the imaging center

When a member expressed a desire to schedule an appointment, our interviewers immediately facilitated a conversation between the member and the imaging center. If the member was reached at a time when the imaging center was closed, the caller asked the member to provide a convenient day and time for the mammogram to be performed. The interviewer then contacted the imaging center on the next business day, scheduled the appointment, and contacted the member.

Reminders and Follow-Up

The callers attempted to contact each member two business days prior to their appointment to remind them of their upcoming mammogram. If that call did not successfully reach the member, a second reminder call was attempted one business day prior to the appointment. After the appointment, the imaging center was contacted to confirm that the member had kept the appointment. If the member failed to show for their appointment, the interviewer attempted to contact the member to determine the reason why. Two outreach calls were attempted for each no-show member.

Results

The intervention was conducted between May and December of 2003. The telephone protocol and the way unsuccessful calls were escalated is shown in Table 15. Of the 505 members who were targeted for outreach, 259 (51.3%) were contacted. The results of this effort are shown in Figure 12.

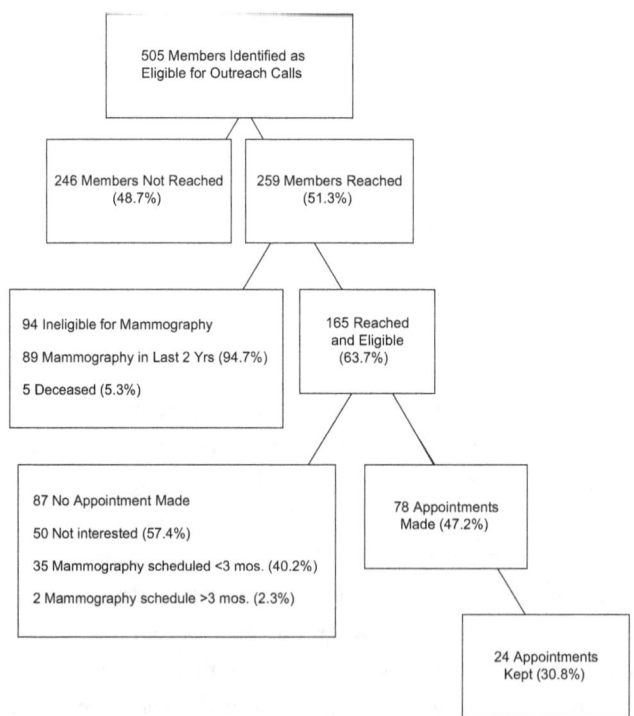

Of the 259 patients contacted, 165 (63.7%) were defined as eligible for mammography. Appointments were made for 78 (47.2%) of these women. 24 (30.8%) of such appointments were actually kept and mammography conducted. Thus, of the initial 505 eligible members, fewer than 5% ultimately obtained a mammogram through the process of this intervention.

87 women refused an appointment. In 50 (57.5%), the person simply was not interested in having a mammogram. 35 (40.2%) members claimed they already had a mammogram scheduled within 3 months, and 2 (2.3%) claimed mammograms had been scheduled in the more distant future. None of these women opted to accept our offer to reschedule an appointment.

Of the 246 members who were defined as not contacted, 78 (31.7%) had disconnected phone numbers. In 81 cases (32.9%), an incorrect phone number was present, and we were unable to find a valid alternative number. The remainder were not contacted due to the phone ringing with a busy signal, the member not being available to speak to the interviewer, or the phone being answered by an answering machine.

Of the 94 women reached but defined as ineligible for mammography, 89 (94.7%) told us that they had undergone a mammogram within the last two years. Further review of these cases indeed revealed a claim in our data system in 41 cases (46%). Five (5.3%) additional members in this category, defined as ineligible, were in fact deceased.

The results of callers' efforts to contact members with appointment reminders revealed that we were successful in only 23 (29.5%) of such reminder calls. Interestingly, despite being contacted shortly before the scheduled study, only seven of the 23 women reminded (30.4%) actually kept their appointment.

Although the percentage of members who kept their appointment tended to be higher within the groups who actually scheduled their appointment close to the time of our initial contact, differences between the 1–10 days group and the 10–<30 days group did not reach statistical significance. (P=.09, odds ratio=2.619 with a confidence interval of [.88, 8.0] inclusive of one.)

To understand why appointments were not kept, the interviewers did attempt to reach members who did not keep their appointments. They were able to reach 17 of the 54 no-show members (31.5%). As shown in Table 16, no single dominant cause could be identified.

Table 16. *Reason given for failing to keep appointment*

Contact: **Members who did not keep their appointment**

Reached 17 of 54 (31.5%)

Reason	Number	Percentage
Sickness	4	23.53%
Personal scheduling conflict	3	17.65%
Could not find site	2	11.76%
Problem at Imaging Center, appointment refused	2	11.76%
Decided to contact PCP	2	11.76%
Lost insurance coverage	1	5.88%
Member refused mammogram - feared compression of breast	1	5.88%
Member changed mind and decided did not want a mammogram	1	5.88%
Member forgot appointment	1	5.88%
TOTALS	**17**	**100.00%**

Discussion

Knowing that mammography saves lives and that access-enhancing interventions improve adherence rates, we attempted to remove an access barrier that we believed to be important for our population by providing, with the member's input, a convenient appointment for mammography.

Several facts from this study are worth emphasizing. We used skilled telephone operators, employees of our own call center who were experienced at talking to patients; they were well trained in the details of this study. We developed a comprehensive escalation of calls to reach these patients, covering all days of the week and all times of the day. Yet despite that, we were able to contact only 51% of the patients. This confirms our findings from other work that attempting to reach patients on the telephone is time-consuming and resource intensive. Indeed, it has been our experience in other situations, such as making appointment reminders and conducting case management follow-up, that reaching patients on the phone is difficult to do.

A further finding was that of those reached, only 63% in fact were eligible for mammography, as the others had already had a mammography or had died. Clearly, there was a large difference between the patients' recollection of having undergone mammography and our administrative data. This calls into question the reliability of using such administrative data for studies such as this. While many may have been telescoping the interval since their last mammogram, as a practical matter, they believed they had already undergone screening, and little we said or did encouraged them to do it again. Finally, and most disappointingly, only 31% of the women for whom we had made an appointment actually kept it. 69% did not. While "sickness" was given as the most common reason, no single cause dominated the reasons for failure to keep the appointment.

These findings also pose important ethical, philosophic, and practical questions. If patients refuse or neglect to show up for their personally scheduled cancer screening or medical evaluation appointments, given that resources for outreach are a scarce and expensive commodity, should providers and health care organizations continue to be held liable for obtaining these tests? Since decisions regarding the expenditure of precious resources must be made strategically, the time might soon come when organizations are increasingly forced to forgo resource intensive interventions that are noble in intent but questionable with respect to efficacy.

The health care industry continues to move in the direction of measuring and comparing quality within and between managed care and provider organizations. Clearly, payers, employers, and the government are looking to incent quality through pay-for-performance programs, such as adherence to HEDIS indicators. While the success of this approach is not yet certain, nevertheless this imperative requires these organizations to expend scarce and expensive resources to meet specific levels of adherence to quality-of-care indicators.

Again, in line with the concerns we raised above, we wonder whether measurement and pay-for-performance systems should take into consideration the efforts of organizations that expend resources but fail to raise adherence rates.

And finally, how much, if at all, should these programs consider the effects of patient behavior on adherence rates of key screening and quality indicators when reporting on and rewarding provider and plan accomplishments?

The View Sixteen Years Later

The mammogram project's low yield despite significant effort precluded widespread implementation. Now in 2019 with new technology, we can imagine a different mode of outreach within a different model of patient and LHS accountability. Assuming the availability of smartphones, we can alert patients through the smartphone of their necessary but as yet unscheduled mammogram and provide an application that will allow them to schedule the mammogram at their convenience. We can imagine a situation where the application will remind them within two weeks of the pending appointment.

Behavioral nudging[35] can be used to improve adherence to guidelines while retaining patient autonomy and personal responsibility. Auditing of LHS mammogram appointment capacity by storing the appointment date requested and dates of offered and ultimately accepted appointments should serve as evidence that the LHS met its HEDIS screening obligation even for patients who do not receive a mammogram. Thus, the patient assumes her part of the responsibility for screening failure rather than foisting the total responsibility on the LHS. The low cost of outreach will obviate the need to punish the nonadherent patient by withholding future screening outreach efforts. However, penalties for no-shows at appointments should be built into future scheduling efforts.

Emergency Room as Canary in the Mines of the Learning Health System

A learning health system has many sites of care delivery, including outpatient offices, surgery centers, urgicenters, dialysis sites, school health care clinics, and emergency rooms.

A common place where activity might detect system failure is the emergency room. Patients who have been unable to gain access to primary care, or who have not been adequately treated, or who have deteriorated in spite of best practice, if they have not died or abandoned the health care delivery system, are ultimately captured in the safety net of the emergency room. Thus, studying the people who are brought to the emergency room and the experience of this safety net site can potentially provide insight into the operational health of the larger health care delivery system.

In days of old, miners would bring canaries into the mines because the canaries were exquisitely sensitive to deadly mine gas. When the canary fell over, the miners knew it was time to evacuate. Similarly, thoughtful surveillance on the activity of the emergency room can be an early warning sign of health system ill health.

How to Assess Emergency Room Overcrowding

Question #1: Over the past three years, has there been a progressive increase in overcrowding in the emergency department?

A direct answer to this would require census data every six hours for the emergency room displayed as a statistical process control chart[36-39] over the years 2016, 2017, and 2018.

Census data is unavailable, but an analytic proxy could be ED dwell time. ED dwell time is defined as the difference in hours between the moment of ED discharge and the moment of ED triage. It is reasonable to assume that if ED dwell time increases, then the actual census population should increase as well.

The complete analysis of the ED program requires a team with focus, local context knowledge, and authority to institute additional project specific data collection efforts. This analysis is a quick and dirty analysis from available data that will provide some clues as to how to maintain surveillance and monitor interventional impact.

Let's first focus on those patients who ultimately are admitted to the hospital. Some in the ED believe that the inability to admit to the hospital because of a too-high occupancy rate causes a "back-up problem" and that if the hospital more efficiently processed its patients and more importantly could open up beds for admission when needed by the ED, the ED could decant and have fewer "dwelling hospitalization-needy patients."

Using Clinical Looking Glass, we can identify all the ED triage patients whose disposition was ultimately admitted. We will restrict ourselves to patients 18 years of age and older and only in the months of January and the end of August in 2016, 2017, and 2018. This analysis was performed when only eight months were available in 2018 to answer the question. The month restriction is to make sure that we have same months for analysis over three years, thereby allowing us to control for seasonal effects. We calculate the dwell time for each patient from triage to hospital admission and then regress on the three years as factors.

```
Coefficients:
                  Estimate Std. Error t value Pr(>|t|)
(Intercept)       10.09781    0.06319  159.81   <2e-16 ***
YearAsFactor2017   1.01006    0.09058   11.15   <2e-16 ***
YearAsFactor2018   1.97268    0.09070   21.75   <2e-16 ***
```

Figure 11. Regression of year on ED dwell time (intercept is mean ED dwell time at baseline 2016)

Interpretation

- The average dwell time in 2016 was 10 hours. In 2015, it was 11 hours, and in 2018, it was 12 hours.
- This 19.5% change from the mean baseline of 2016 is highly significant.
- Result: the dwell time has consistently worsened for admitted patients from 2016 to the present.

For those interested, we provide a statistical process control chart summarizing the mean dwell time by month grouped by year (Figure 12).

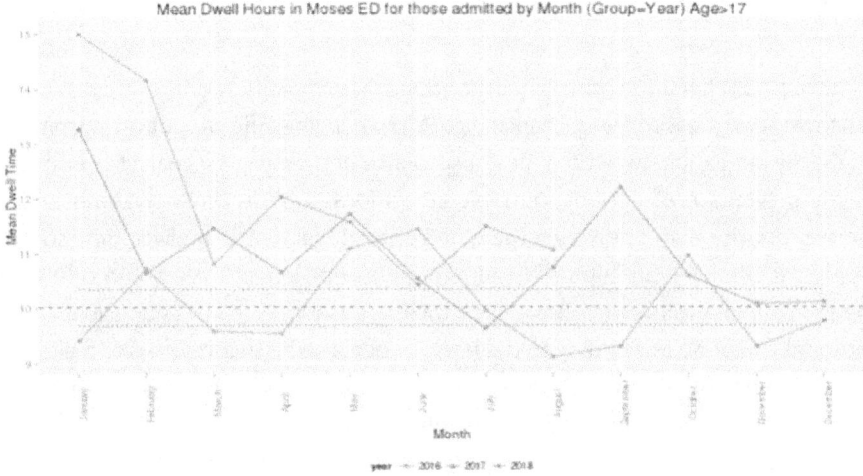

Figure 12. Mean ED dwell time by month grouped by year (statistical process control chart)

As you can see, the 2018 line ends at August because at the time of the analysis, there was no information for the full month of September 2018. For seven of the eight months of 2018, 2018 has a longer dwell time than 2016.

A tabular representation of the graphic is provided in Table 17.

Table 17. Mean ED dwell time by month grouped by year

Number of Hours from triage to Admission Patients Greater than or equal to 18			
	2016	2017	2018
January	9.4	13.3	15
February	10.7	10.7	14
March	9.6	11.5	10.8
April	9.5	10.7	12
May	11.1	11.7	11.6
June	11.4	10.5	10.4
July	10	9.6	11.5
August	9.1	10.7	11

Question #2: What is the cause of the increasing dwell time?
There are two areas of focus: changing goals or changing efficiency of the hospital or ED. Is the increasing dwell time the consequence of changing ED goals? For example, is the prevention of non-reimbursable admissions, such as one-day admissions, a greater priority than optimizing the siloed operational metric of dwell time so that some patients who are ultimately admitted are kept longer than would otherwise be the case in a vain effort to preclude their admission? The ED, as an agent of the hospital, might be responding to the hospital demanding that it serves as a filter for non-reimbursable admissions exhausting every effort possible to preclude an unnecessary admission, thereby backing up its operation.

A second area of focus could be the availability of efflux into the hospital itself. If the hospital had closed beds physically or functionally reduced beds by blocking them with an increased length of stay caused by operational inefficiencies, this efflux problem could back up the ED, thus creating the observed increased dwell time.

Teasing out these issues would require a team with the extra on-the-ground, real-time collection of information.

Question #3: Is there evidence of increasing patient complexity?
Is there evidence of increased patient complexity causing a reduction of throughput by burdening staff so they cannot efficiently process patients and open up hospital beds?

This is somewhat difficult to answer as this hospital—like others nationally—has made efforts to improve financial collections by improving code capture. This has the undesirable analytic effect of making it possible that any billing code comorbidity increase might be reflective of coding artifact rather than patient attribute change.[40] However, it behooves us to take a look at the data as it is while keeping in mind this proviso.

There are two ways to look at the question of care intensity as it impacts bed availability:

1. Look at the 3m APR DRG weight. Each patient admitted is given a 3M diagnosis with a weight assigned to that admission. The weight is supposedly an approximation of the effort required to care for admissions with this APR diagnostic category.

2. Look at the 3M APR DRG average LOS. This is a metric that assigns to each admission the expected national average LOS. While it may be that the "Bronx is different" (a usual refrain that I will not address here), it could still be a consistent estimator of change.

Let's consider the DRG weight approach.

Using Clinical Looking Glass, we find that the APR DRG weight increased by 9% from 2016 to 2018.

To demonstrate this 9% worsening of APR DRG weight, first regress APR DRG Weight on Year (Figure 13).

```
Coefficients:
              Estimate Std. Error t value Pr(>|t|)
(Intercept)  1.56369    0.01405  111.329  < 2e-16  ***
dcYear2017   0.08635    0.02001    4.316 1.59e-05  ***
dcYear2018   0.14468    0.02146    6.743 1.57e-11  ***
---
Signif. codes:  0 '***' 0.001 '**' 0.01 '*' 0.05 '.' 0.1 ' ' 1
```

Figure 13. Regression DRG weight upon year

We find that the average APR DRG weight in 2016 was 1.56. The additional DRG weight from the 2016 value is .144. So .144/1.56 is the percent increase in DRG weight or 9%. Keep in mind the ED dwell time went up 20% (2/10).

Now let's consider how the 3M APR DRG LOS adjuster believes this increase in DRG weight should have impacted the LOS.

We first regress the average LOS APR DRG on patient year of admission.

```
Coefficients:
            Estimate Std. Error t value Pr(>|t|)
(Intercept)  5.13489    0.02883 178.097  < 2e-16 ***
dcYear2017   0.02295    0.04107   0.559 0.576214
dcYear2018   0.14674    0.04404   3.332 0.000864 ***
---

Signif. codes:  0 '****' 0.001 '***' 0.01 '**' 0.05 '.' 0.1 ' ' 1
```

Figure 14. Regress APR DRG length of stay expected by year

We find at baseline 2016, 3M predicted a LOS average for our patient mix of 5.13 days. In the year 2018, it anticipated an increase of .14 days in average LOS. This makes for a 2.8% (.146/5.13) expected increase in average LOS.

Table 18. Discharges by month and year of discharge from Moses, age 18

	2016	2017	2018	Sum	Per cent
January	3097	3100	3146	9343	12.17
February	3122	2851	2974	8947	11.65
March	3475	3229	2915	9619	12.52
April	3253	3076	3271	9600	12.5
May	3247	3233	3512	9992	13.01
June	3127	3224	3309	9660	12.58
July	3106	3197	3368	9671	12.59
August	3148	3297	3522	9967	12.98
Sum	25575	25207	26017	76799	100

Overall, we have an increase in expected hospital bed usage 3M APR DRG average length of stay of 2.8% and an increase in total number of discharges of 1.7%. The extent to which the increase in discharges and increase in intensity in an already-burdened inpatient service functionally blocks ED discharge needs to be considered. Perhaps there is a theoretic target hospital vacancy required to assure efficient hospital performance to process patients and open up beds.

Question #4: Is there evidence of increasing nonadmitted ED patient workload?
Do we have evidence from nonadmitted patients of increased workload of the ED that could degrade its ability to process people expeditiously?

Here we look at nonadmitted ED patients in the three years of interest.

Table 19. ED Moses non-admitted with both triage and discharge date time Jan–Aug

	2016	2017	2018	Sum	Per cent
January	23689	24970	24178	72837	13.6
February	23662	19820	22824	66306	12.38
March	25847	21154	20855	67856	12.67
April	23208	21472	20561	65241	12.18
May	23738	22807	23212	69757	13.02
June	22069	21241	20818	64128	11.97
July	22067	21315	21420	64802	12.1
August	22344	21130	21248	64722	12.08
Sum	186624	173909	175116	535649	100
Per cent	34.84	32.47	32.69	100	100

The table above counted the number of people seen in the ED but not admitted with both a triage and a discharge date:Time. (a 2% volume drop in 2018 compared to 2016).

Here we look at the statistical process control chart[36-39] of the throughput mean for the nonadmitted:

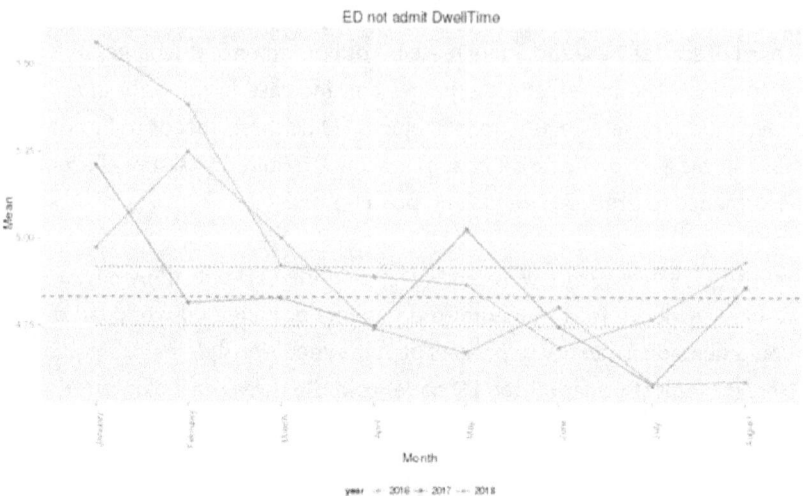

Figure 15. Mean dwell time of nonadmitted ED Moses patients by month and year

We convert this to tabular form.

Table 20. Mean dwell time for ED non-admitted patients

Years Month	2016	2017	2018	Grand Total
January	5.0	5.2	5.6	5.3
February	5.2	4.8	5.4	5.2
March	5.0	4.8	4.9	4.9
April	4.7	4.7	4.9	4.8
May	4.7	5.0	4.9	4.9
June	4.8	4.7	4.7	4.7
July	4.6	4.6	4.8	4.6
August	4.6	4.9	4.9	4.8
Grand Total	**4.8**	**4.9**	**5.0**	**4.9**

We see that 2018 had 2/10 of an hour longer dwell time in 2018 than 2016, an increase of 4%.

Table 21. Regressing dwell time on year

```
Coefficients:
            Estimate Std. Error t value Pr(>|t|)
(Intercept)  4.83311   0.02241  215.656  < 2e-16  ***
year2017     0.02845   0.03227    0.882    0.378
year2018     0.18158   0.03221    5.637 1.73e-08  ***
---
Signif. codes:  0 '***' 0.001 '**' 0.01 '*' 0.05 '.' 0.1 ' ' 1
```

Average dwell time for ED visits at Moses that were not admitted in 2016 was 4.8 hours. In 2018, the average increase was .18 hours more and was statistically significant.

Question #5: Are there operational insights to be gained by studying the time of ED triage for those ultimately admitted to the hospital?
It is sometimes suspected that delays in processing patients can be linked to a specific time when staffing is particularly low either in the ED or in the hospital. If only we could see the activity on a 24-hour clock, we might get some insight on where the problem lies. On a 24-hour clock, the following occurs:

You really do not get much insight from a review of patient volume by hour alone.

You must focus on the issue of interest—mean dwell time in the ED by triage hour of the day for those ultimately admitted. In fact, you might suspect that day of the week as well as hour of the day might be revealing of operational differences. Rather than analyzing by the individual day of the week, we consider days of the week that have similar characteristics in terms of staffing. We study weekdays (Monday, Tuesday, Wednesday, and Thursday) and weekend days (Saturday and Sunday). Friday is an intermediate day and will be ignored in the analysis.

Restricting our interest to patients over age 40 who were evaluated in ED triage and then admitted to Moses (N=2,865) in May 2018, we look first at the percentiles of ED dwell time hours by day of week (Table 24).

Table 22. Number of admissions from ED by triage hour of day by year

	2016	2017	2018	Sum	Per cent
00	1720	1641	1184	4545	5.95
01	1306	1316	924	3546	4.64
02	1119	1040	744	2903	3.8
03	964	863	588	2415	3.16
04	855	703	558	2116	2.77
05	1018	914	685	2617	3.43
06	1123	1067	802	2992	3.92
07	743	701	619	2063	2.7
08	627	539	405	1571	2.06
09	442	449	316	1207	1.58
10	392	438	284	1114	1.46
11	430	425	289	1144	1.5
12	490	463	308	1261	1.65
13	532	538	381	1451	1.9
14	599	680	420	1699	2.22
15	1082	1142	687	2911	3.81
16	1450	1473	890	3813	4.99
17	1727	1771	997	4495	5.88
18	2102	2023	1243	5368	7.03
19	2199	2077	1390	5666	7.42
20	2140	2000	1220	5360	7.02
21	2042	1999	1403	5444	7.13
22	2139	1986	1288	5413	7.08
23	2097	1942	1251	5290	6.92
Sum	29338	28190	18876	76404	100
Per cent	38.4	36.9	24.71	100	100

Table 23. Column percent admitted from Moses ED by triage hour of day by year

hour ▾	2016	2017	2018
0	5.86%	5.82%	6.27%
1	4.45%	4.67%	4.90%
2	3.81%	3.69%	3.94%
3	3.29%	3.06%	3.12%
4	2.91%	2.49%	2.96%
5	3.47%	3.24%	3.63%
6	3.83%	3.79%	4.25%
7	2.53%	2.49%	3.28%
8	2.14%	1.91%	2.15%
9	1.51%	1.59%	1.67%
10	1.34%	1.55%	1.50%
11	1.47%	1.51%	1.53%
12	1.67%	1.64%	1.63%
13	1.81%	1.91%	2.02%
14	2.04%	2.41%	2.23%
15	3.69%	4.05%	3.64%
16	4.94%	5.23%	4.71%
17	5.89%	6.28%	5.28%
18	7.16%	7.18%	6.59%
19	7.50%	7.37%	7.36%
20	7.29%	7.09%	6.46%
21	6.96%	7.09%	7.43%
22	7.29%	7.05%	6.82%
23	7.15%	6.89%	6.63%
(blank)	0.00%	0.00%	0.00%
Grand Total	100.00%	100.00%	100.00%

Table 24. Dwell time in hours by percentile by day of week

Percentile	5th	10th	25th	Median	75th	90th	95th
Mon–Thurs	3.7	4.5	6.4	9.2	13.1	21	26
Sat–Sun	2.6	3.5	4.2	5.7	11.3	15.7	20.3

Below, we look at the same data in a Statistical Process Control chart plotting the mean dwell time by hour of day separately for weekdays and weekends (Figure 16).

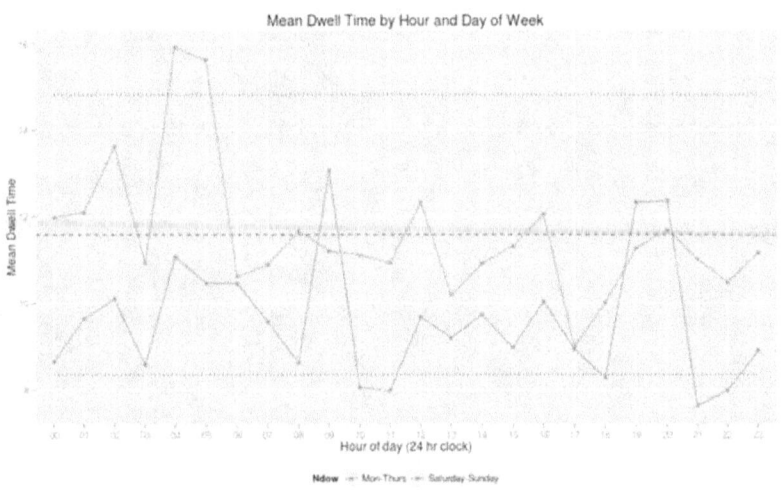

Mean Dwell Time by Hour and Day of Week

Figure 16. Mean dwell time by hour and week/weekend day at Moses for ≥40-year-olds in May 2018

This Process Control Chart clearly shows that weekday admissions take longer to be admitted than weekend admissions for 21 of the 24 hours in a day. This is only the beginning of the analysis.

The purpose of this chapter is to demonstrate that even with all the data and analytic rigor providing surveillance markers for the problem and a detailed clock description of system behavior, you still cannot tell *why* patients are not admitted earlier. *Why* are they languishing in the emergency room? For that sort of analysis, we must engage a PDCA cycle shadowing the participants in the emergency room and learning what is delaying their diagnostic decisions. Once they make the decision to admit, what is delaying the transfer to the hospital bed? Contemporaneously, there needs to be an assessment on the hospital side of what is delaying the opening of the room that is ultimately opened up for the admission—Delayed discharge orders? Meds? Transportation? Cleaning of the room? This level of detail is not available in the EMR, and defined people must engage collaboratively with the clinicians and staff in both the ER and the hospital floor (at the gemba) in real time to find the relevant issues and possible solutions. Where you don't find this effort, you have discovered the footprint of missing management.

Appropriate Outpatient Management of Patients Might Preclude Unnecessary Emergency Department Visits

---

Problem: The health care delivery system owns outpatient capacity, emergency department services, and inpatient beds. A careful study of the system reveals an emergency room with intolerable delays overburdened with a huge census at any time, which compromises efficiency. It is hypothesized that some of the emergency room census could be prevented by improving outpatient access and service quality in the outpatient universe. How might one begin to analyze this question and assess the potential contribution of inadequate outpatient service to the overburdening of the emergency room? A system view considers all the available assets and sets a goal optimizing the use of those assets to achieve the goal.[41,42]

Formulate the Answerable Question

For patients in a primary care relationship with our system, do we have evidence that they are using the ED inappropriately? The implication of inappropriate use is that we are not addressing the patient's clinical needs in the appropriate outpatient setting, which forces them to come to the emergency department for care.

1. Are these visits preventable?
2. Quantitate the unnecessary burden these patients are placing on ED operations.

The question will be actualized with the following case definitions:

1. Adult population: age≥21.
2. Patients in a relationship with Montefiore: any patient with at least one outpatient visit in one of our primary care medical groups in 2017. We will consider definitional modifications later. The notion is that if you are in a primary care relationship, we can teach you to have expectations of us to deliver care in the appropriate setting.
3. Evaluate Moses ED use in May 2018 for potentially preventable ED visits.

Out of the individuals who had emergency room visits, which visits resulted in a discharge to home rather than in admission? We will make the first-order assumption that within this group are a large number of preventable ED visits.

Clinical Looking Glass Considerations

We will be using an event collection because we seek all emergency room visits belonging to the eligible group of patients. The object of analysis is the ED triage patient visit. The same patient can be considered multiple times as each ED visit has the potential for prevention.

The first order of business is to create a condition line that will restrict the analysis to those patients in a relationship with us. We have decided to use a single visit in 2017 in the medical group as evidence of a relationship. You can, of course, require more than one visit in future analyses. A snapshot of this list of MMG primary care clinics is provided below.

The first condition line should be of adults aged ≥21 in the year 2017 who had an outpatient visit at one of the 24 specific sites from our list. You will note that while the event collection will ultimately be "All" and point to emergency room triages, the first line qualifies the patients as belonging to the primary care outpatient population. We will use the earliest outpatient visit in 2017 in one of these MMG outpatient clinics as the indicator variable of a Montefiore relationship.

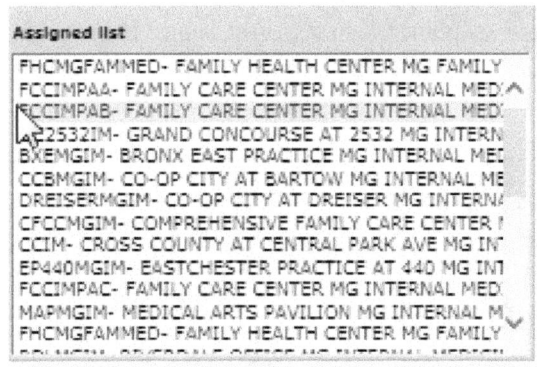

Figure 17. Sample of clinics in the set of primary care medical group

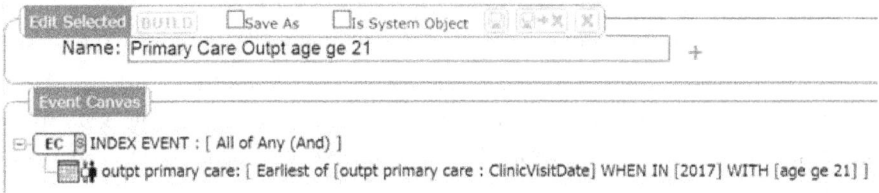

Figure 18. Primary care patients aged ≥21 MMG in 2017

In 2017, 146,423 people who were aged ≥21 were seen in the MMG primary care clinic at least once. Now find those who had an ED visit in the month of May 2018 in the Moses Emergency Department.

Build the second condition line by choosing "All" and defining the event by "ED triage."

Now define two ED attributes: one for facility (Moses) and one for disposition (discharged to home).

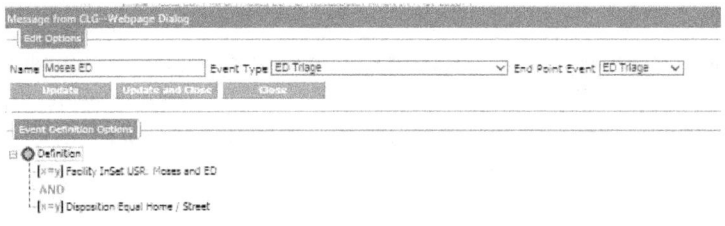

Figure 19: ED visit attributes Moses and disposition to home

On the event canvas point the Index Event line to the ED visits so when you browse the collection, you will be able to count all the ED visits and see all their attributes.

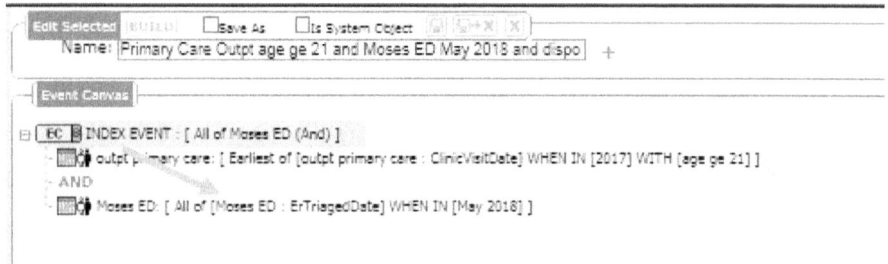

Figure 20. ED visits for patients who had a Montefiore relationship

We note that in May 2018, there were 1,625 emergency room visits in the Moses ED for patients ultimately discharged to home who had a relationship with the MMG medical group. Let's contextualize this. How many emergency room triage visits from the medical group were in Moses in May 2018? Consider all ED triage visits, not just those discharged to home.

Build the event collection to see how many visits to the ED (do not restrict to Discharge to Home because you want to see how much total business there is in the ED).

Remove disposition=home.

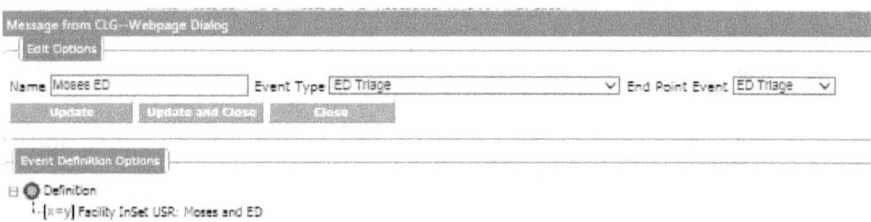

What we see is a snapshot of our total business in the ED by active medical group Montefiore patients (N=2,637). Of the 2,637 ED visits, 1,625 of them were discharged to home and not admitted. This means that approximately 62% of the medical group ED visits in May 2018 might have been preventable.

What percent of all Moses ED visits in the month of May were caused by potentially preventable medical group triage events?

We are now asking the following question: Of the total work product of the Moses ED, what percent could have been prevented by removing the medical group preventables?

We will count the total number of ED visits to the Moses ED without requiring a disposition of home and without requiring prior evidence of a Montefiore relationship (Figure 21).

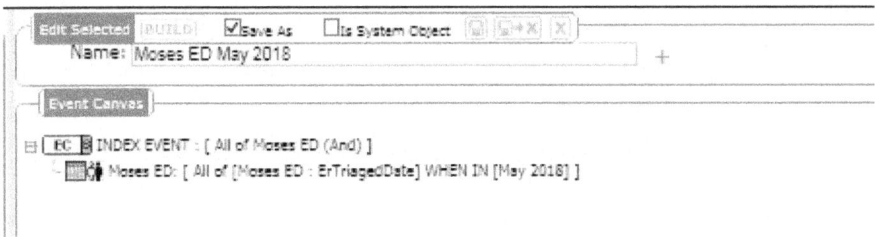

Figure 21. All Moses ED visits in May 2018

Browse the ED collection to build the table of dispositions and then pivot on the disposition.

Give us the total number of ED triage visits in the Moses ED in May 2018, and provide the breakdown of the disposition for those visits in a pivot.

Table 25. Disposition of ED visits at Moses in May 2018

Disposition	Count
Home/Street	9,736
Inpatient Admission	2,865
BLANK	725
Eloped	428
UNKNOWN	144
Nursing Home	85
Other	24
Expired	15
Send to L&D	2
(blank)	
Grand Total	14,024

Of the 14,024 visits to Moses, the proportion of preventable admissions from the medical group is 1.625/14,024 or 11.5% of Moses's ED volume in May.

The case definition for the presence of a Montefiore relationship was based upon an outpatient visit to the primary care clinic in 2017. We can alter the definition to include a primary care clinic visit in the 1–365 days before the ED visit. Or we can further broaden the definition by including any outpatient visit, not just an outpatient visit to the primary care clinic. The use of any outpatient visit implies that we should be teaching our patients at every outpatient encounter that there are alternatives to the emergency department and that any ED visit that results in an ultimate disposition to home is a system failure.

Table 26 provides the counts of preventable ED visits by type of encounter establishing a Montefiore relationship and the time window in which that encounter took place. I also provide the percent of the May 2018 Moses ED total visits for which these visits are responsible.

Table 26. Count of ED patients discharged to home by type and time of previous outpatient encounter (% of total ED count), May 2018

Type of Encounter	Time of At least Once in 2017	Previous Encounter At least Once 1–365 days before
MMG Primary Care	1,625 (11.5%)	1,925 (13.5%)
Any Outpatient Activity	2,930 (20.6%)	5,392 (38%)

Clearly, there is an opportunity to intervene and reduce the work burden of the emergency room.

However, one should, at this time, be a little cautious. Not all people sent home were inappropriate ED visits. Consider those patients who required the resources of an emergency room to rule out a more serious problem.

Looking at the leading diagnoses of these emergency room visits (Table 27), you find chest pain, calculus of kidney, and epigastric pain. It is not too much of a stretch to suspect that the unique capabilities and resources of the emergency room were necessary to determine the benign nature of these complaints. What is missing from the first-order disposition to home analysis is the workup and treatment provided while in the ED. For example, one might conclude that, if the patient required Intravenous medication and/or fluids, an emergent CT scan, serial cardiac markers, laceration repair, incision and drainage of an abscess, Foley placement, splinting, or

Table 27. Primary diagnoses ED visits discharged to home in sort order (sample)

Primary Diagnosis	Count
R07.9-Chest pain, unspecified	166
R42-Dizziness and giddiness	131
M54.5-Low back pain	117
R51-Headache	95
J45.901-Unspecified asthma with (acute) exacerbation	64
N39.0-Urinary tract infection, site not specified	60
R07.89-Other chest pain	59
R10.13-Epigastric pain	52
J06.9-Acute upper respiratory infection, unspecified	51
R05-Cough	48
M54.2-Cervicalgia	41
J45.909-Unspecified asthma, uncomplicated	41
K52.9-Noninfective gastroenteritis and colitis, unspecified	39
J02.9-Acute pharyngitis, unspecified	37
R06.02-Shortness of breath	36
R21-Rash and other nonspecific skin eruption	35
M25.561-Pain in right knee	33
R10.9-Unspecified abdominal pain	33
M25.562-Pain in left knee	33
R00.2-Palpitations	29
N20.0-Calculus of kidney	29

another procedure, the ED visit was necessary even if the patient was ultimately discharged to home instead of admitted.

The most reliable way to determine which ED visits are unnecessary is to ask the ED doctor. By providing a list of capabilities expected of the outpatient facilities with which the patient has a relationship, the emergency department doctor can contemporaneously record whether the clinical scenario he just reviewed should have been managed at the home clinic. An engaged ED doctor providing feedback to the home clinic can support an effective PDSA cycle.

Of the 1,625 ED visits for patients discharged to home and seen in 2017 in an MMG outpatient clinic, the following occurred:

- 273 ED visits had an MMG clinic visit within the antecedent 14 days.
- 374 ED visits had an MMG clinic visit within the antecedent 21 days.
- 443 ED visits had an MMG clinic visit within the antecedent 28 days (Figure 22).

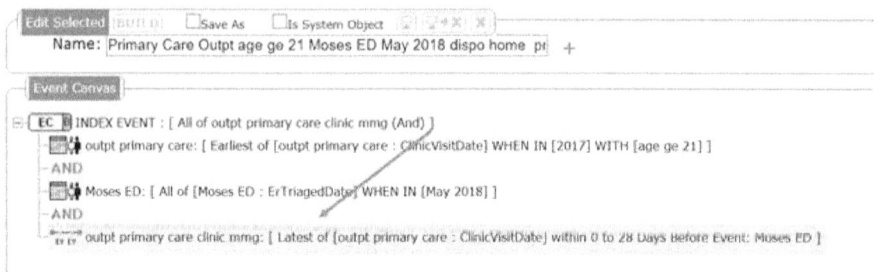

Figure 22. ED visits of Montefiore patients in May 2018 discharged to home with an antecedent MMG outpatient visit (0–28 days)

To determine which of the ED visits could have been prevented if, in the antecedent clinic visit, some intervention for an active problem then recognizable had been undertaken requires the subtlety of a clinician performing a chart review. To get a sense of how much work this would entail for each clinic, I consider the number of charts for review per clinic if we demanded that each clinic reviewed their patients with an ED visit to Moses discharged to home in May 2018 (Table 28).

Table 28. Count of outpatient encounters in the 30 days antecedent to a Moses ED visit, May 2018, needing review

Outpatient Clinic (Department)	Count
GRAND CONCOURSE AT 2532 MG INTERNAL MEDICINE-GC2532IM	66
MEDICAL ARTS PAVILION MG INTERNAL MEDICINE-MAPMGIM	56
FAMILY HEALTH CENTER MG FAMILY MEDICINE-FHCMGFAMMED	53
COMPREHENSIVE HEALTH CARE CENTER MG INTERNAL MEDICINE-CHCCMGIM	41

FAMILY CARE CENTER MG INTERNAL MEDICINE - PAC-FCCIMPAC	36
WILLIAMSBRIDGE PRACTICE AT 3011 MG FAMILY MEDICINE-WLMSMGFAMMED	29
FAMILY CARE CENTER MG INTERNAL MEDICINE - PAA-FCCIMPAA	26
FAMILY CARE CENTER MG INTERNAL MEDICINE - PAB-FCCIMPAB	24
UNIVERSITY AVENUE FAMILY PRACTICE MG INTERNAL MEDICINE-UNIVMGIM	23
BRONX EAST PRACTICE MG INTERNAL MEDICINE-BXEMGIM	22
MARBLE HILL FAMILY PRACTICE MG INTERNAL MEDICINE-MRBLMGIM	11
CO-OP CITY AT BARTOW MG INTERNAL MEDICINE-CCBMGIM	11
WEST FARMS FAMILY PRACTICE MG FAMILY MEDICINE-WFFPMGFAMMED	9
VIA VERDE MG FAMILY MEDICINE-VVMGFAMMED	8
CROSS COUNTY AT CENTRAL PARK AVE MG INTERNAL MEDICINE-CCIM	6
RIVERDALE OFFICE MG INTERNAL MEDICINE-RDLMGIM	6
COMPREHENSIVE FAMILY CARE CENTER MG INTERNAL MEDICINE-CFCCMGIM	5
CASTLE HILL FAMILY PRACTICE MG FAMILY MEDICINE-CSTLMGFAMPLA	4
UNIVERSITY AVENUE FAMILY PRACTICE MG FAMILY MEDICINE-UNIVMGFAMMED	3
CO-OP CITY AT DREISER MG INTERNAL MEDICINE-DREISERMGIM	2
EASTCHESTER PRACTICE AT 440 MG INTERNAL MEDICINE-EP440MGIM	1
WILLIAMSBRIDGE PRACTICE AT 3011 MG INTERNAL MEDICINE-WLLFPIM	1
(blank)	
Grand Total	**443**

The clinic could identify systematic failures to provide timely access for evolving knowable problems as well as access for unexpected new onset issues.

We have focused on the emergency room visits in which the patient was discharged to go home, but the clinics could also focus, if they wished, upon those admitted to explore what opportunities they had to prevent such deterioration. Obviously, the more proximal in time the outpatient visit, the more reasonable it is to assume that the problem was manifest and potentially remediable.

The ability to create cohorts in a timely manner to support a PDSA cycle can radically transform the cultural notions of clinical ownership by the clinics of their patients, with targeted interventions to improve their performance.

Another idea, offered by an ED colleague David Esses, might be to use the acuity level (Table 29) as the starting point. For example, many acuity-level Nonurgent visits are avoidable. As you go up the acuity scale (down in numbers) to Semiurgent and

Urgent, the percentage of avoidable visits decreases regardless of ultimate disposition to home or hospital.

Table 29: Priority of ED visits discharged to home in May 2018 in patients seen by MMG clinic in 2017

Priority	Count	PCT	Cumulative PCT
Nonurgent	68	4%	4%
Semiurgent	673	42%	46%
Urgent	676	42%	88%
Emergent	196	12%	100%

Does a Learning Health System Need EMR Data, or Is Administrative Data Enough? The Case of the Dehydrated Patient

The learning health system considers patient groups whose complicated care can lead to iatrogenic complications, and the system seeks to prevent them. One such group includes cancer patients who present to our emergency room for care after chemotherapy. Among the causes includes dehydration due to nausea and vomiting, a consequence of the chemotherapy.

The aim of this exercise is to determine patients who received chemotherapy resulting in an ED visit for dehydration. While the corrective for this might include better antiemetic therapy or the availability of patient navigators that the patient can call for assistance should they begin to experience nausea and vomiting or need IV rehydration, the first step in this analytic process is to establish the extent of the problem as it will determine the sort of resources that can be committed to spare unnecessary expenses.

We will create the chemotherapy set from First Data Bank hierarchical classification used in Clinical Looking Glass.

To establish the extent of the problem, we need to build a cohort identifying all those cancer chemotherapy patients who ended up being evaluated in the ED at least once within 30 days of their chemotherapy in the year 2018 (Figure 23).

1.   Patients receiving chemotherapy drugs (as part of either inpatient or out-patient treatment)
2.   Patients found in the tumor registry in the 10 years prior to chemotherapy
3.   ED triage that occurred within 30 days of the chemotherapy

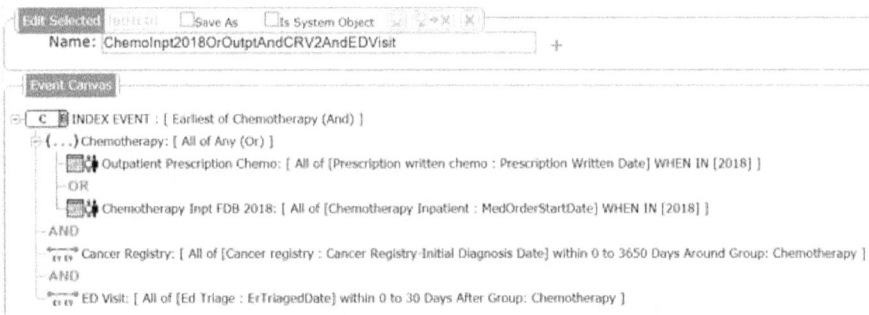

Figure 23. Cancer patients receiving cancer chemotherapy in 2018 and admitted to the ED within 30 days of chemotherapy

The year 2018 cohort contains 1,119 patients who received chemotherapy as part of outpatient or inpatient treatment, were in the cancer registry in the surrounding 10 years (before or after), and had an ED visit within 30 days after either the med order or prescription-written chemotherapy.

Now we want to know how many ED visits are associated with the chemotherapy agents given in 2018 to cancer patients who are found within the registry within 10 years of their chemotherapy.

Notice that we now build an event collection as we want to find all the relevant triage emergency room visits. We change the index event line to have the notion of all and point to the ED visit condition line (Figure 24).

There are 1,966 ED visits among patients who received chemotherapy in 2018 and were in the cancer registry within 10 years of the medication being given.

Now browse the event collection and pivot on disposition to determine whether their ED visit resulted in an admission (Table 30).

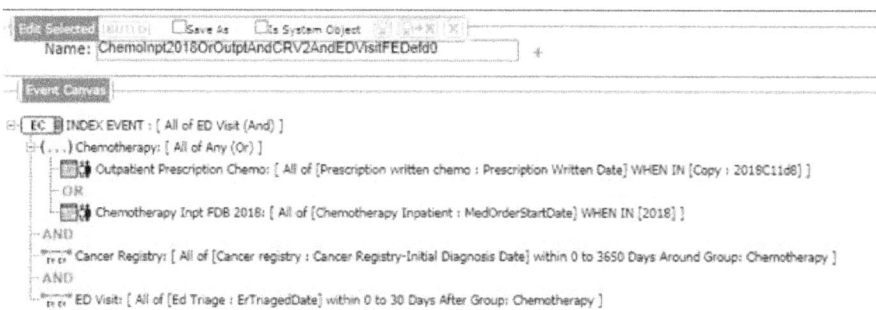

Figure 24. All ED visits within 30 days after chemotherapy given in 2018 in patients in the Tumor Registry

Table 30. Disposition of ED visits within 30 days of receiving chemotherapy

Disposition	Count of disposition
Inpatient Admission	1187
Home / Street	688
UNKNOWN	21
Eloped	20
BLANK	19
Other	16
Expired	11
Nursing Home	2
(blank)	
Grand Total	1964

Now we will look at those who had a diagnosis of dehydration during their ED visit.

Use the event type "ICD Diagnosis" and create the set of dehydration diagnostic codes, and then build a condition line that demands that the dehydration diagnosis occurs during the ED visit. Using the "when in" durational operator pointing to the ED condition line achieves this goal.[3]

There are 141 ED visits with a diagnosis of dehydration by the ICD billing code.

When we browse the data and view the encounter, all of the 141 visits resulted in an admission.

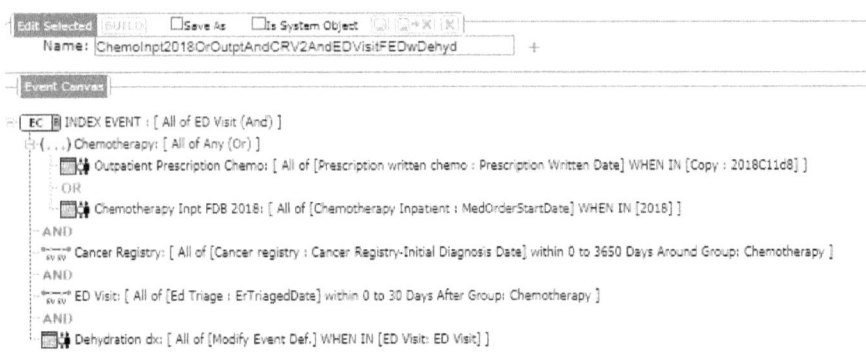

Figure 25. Dehydration ICD diagnosis in ED

Now let us use a clinical data case definition for dehydration, not an administrative billing code. Find those patients whose urine concentration was so high that it was diagnostic of dehydration, a urine-specific gravity greater than or equal to 1.020 during the ED visit (Figure 26).

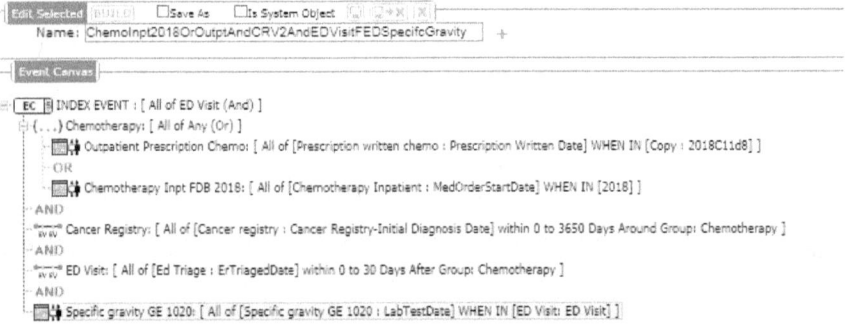

Figure 26. ED visits for chemotherapy patients with a urine-specific gravity greater than or equal to 1020 during the ED stay

There are 203 ED visits with dehydration detected by urine-specific gravity case definition.

Compared with the administrative data ICD code case definition for dehydration, the clinical definition detected 44% more ED visits (203/141=144%).

We should not be surprised that a clinical definition would be more sensitive than a billing code. Billing codes are recorded when higher revenue is to be expected.

Without a revenue-enhancement imperative, there is no reason for the ICD coder to include a diagnosis.

Find the disposition for each ED admission with a urine-specific gravity above 1.020.

Table 31. ED disposition for chemotherapy patients with clinical case definition for dehydration

Disposition in ED (urine-specific gravity)	Count
Inpatient Admission	160
Home / Street	40
UNKNOWN	2
Other	1
(blank)	
Grand Total	**203**

160/203=79% of patients were admitted to the hospital after their ED visit with a urine-specific gravity at 1.020 or above.

Now find the disposition of those with a diagnosis of dehydration based upon the ICD diagnosis code (Table 32).

Table 32. ED disposition for chemotherapy patients with dehydration diagnosed by ICD criteria

Disposition from ED (dehydration)	Count
Inpatient Admission	134
(blank)	
Grand Total	**134**

All patients diagnosed with dehydration ICD-9 were admitted (134 out of 134).

Dehydration diagnosed by specific gravity resulted in an additional 20 admissions, while an additional 40 were diagnosed as dehydrated and returned home, and three had an unknown status.

To obtain a sense of the temporal change in the number of ED visits attributable to chemotherapy-induced dehydration, we merely change the dates in the event collection with the resulting information.

Table 33. Number of ED visits of chemotherapy patients with dehydration by year

Year	Number with specific gravity proven dehydration
2018	203
2017	382
2016	450
2015	455

We see a persistent reduction over the last three years of potentially chemotherapy-induced emergency department dehydration visits, perhaps suggesting better antiemetic management.

Just one more thought. This conclusion assumes that every cancer patient seen in the emergency department had their urine collected or at least that the same proportion of those people were tested in each of the four years. Looking at this question, we find from 2018–2015, 469, 834, 854, and 916 ED visits, respectively, with a urine test with specific gravity. The number of times dehydration could be evaluated by a urine-specific gravity test has declined over the past four years. We therefore cannot be sure without additional information that the absolute number reduction of dehydrated urines supports our conclusion of improved dehydration control. As I promised in the introduction, my purpose in this book is not to complete an analysis but to give you the intuition and understanding to approach extracting meaning from data.

Evaluation of Palliative Care Adequacy for Cancer Patients

N ationally, it is recognized that the timeliness of the provision of palliative care in oncology is abysmal.

Consultation ideally should be at the onset of grave illness with terminal propensity to assure that the wishes of the patient are fully understood and respected. Unfortunately, in many cases, a palliative care consult is provided but five days before death as a required entrance ticket to terminal hospice care. The appropriate use of palliation is earlier in the course when futility is all but obvious, and the patient's physical, spiritual, and social well-being should become the priority. A learning health system should evaluate the timeliness of palliative care for their cancer patient population both from ethical and cost-containment considerations.

Method

We will create a reasonable metric and see how well we perform in providing palliative care consultation—the first step in providing meaningful palliative care.

Create a cohort of cancer patients who died during a hospitalization at Montefiore, and then evaluate their penultimate hospitalization for evidence of a palliative care consult during that penultimate hospitalization or at any time before that hospitalization.

First, find those who were diagnosed with cancer (during any encounter) during 2017. Looking at patients with an ICD diagnosis of malignancy at some point in 2017 (Figure 27), we see this.

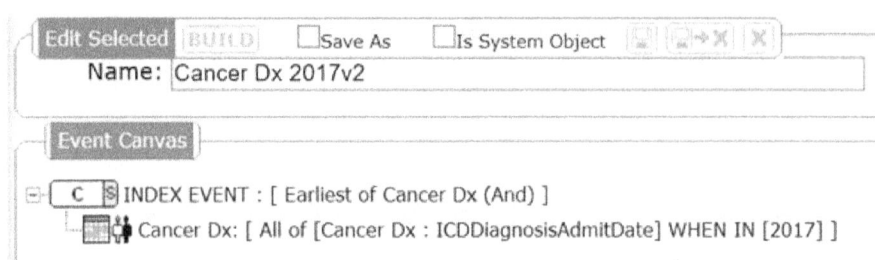

Figure 27. Cancer diagnosis in 2017 (N=28,786)

Now, find those who died during a hospitalization during 2017 by adding a second condition line that represents that hospitalization and require that the disposition=expired. Use the event "inpatient admission" to define the hospitalization.

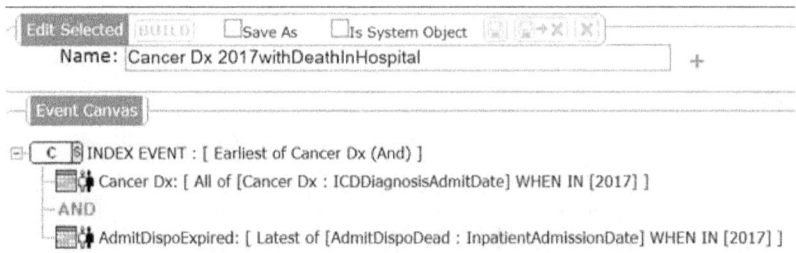

Figure 28. Inpatient admission with disposition=expired

Build the cohort.

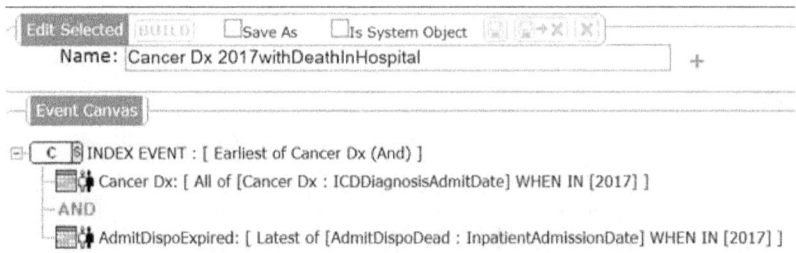

Figure 29. Cancer patients within hospital death in 2017 (N=731)

Now we want to find those with a penultimate hospitalization within 180 days of the hospitalization in which death occurred (death hospitalization).

We will look for the last discharge 0–180 days prior to the hospitalization in which the patient died.

Add a new condition line, and add the hospitalization event to be temporally related 0–180 days before and choose "latest" so we can get the most proximal hospitalization to the death hospitalization and be able to identify the primary diagnoses in that penultimate hospitalization.

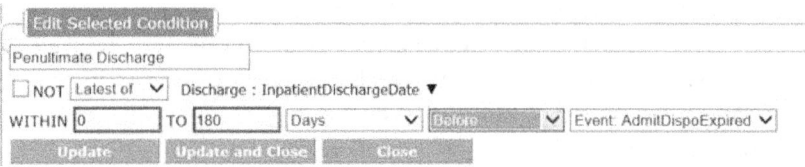

Figure 30. Penultimate discharge: discharge before admission in which patient died

Build the cohort.

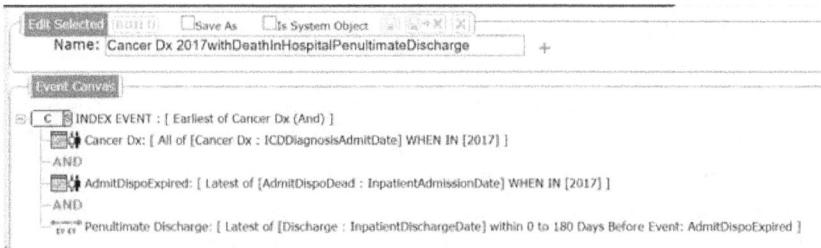

Figure 31. Cancer patients with penultimate discharge prior to admission with death in 2017 (N=480).

The top 65% of cancer ICD diagnoses in this cohort is given in the table below (Table 34).

Table 34. Top 65% of ICD cancer diagnoses in 415 cancer patients with an in-hospital death in 2017 and a penultimate discharge 0–180 days before death hospitalization

ICD Cancer Code	Count
Z85.3: Personal history of malignant neoplasm of breast	31
Z85.46: Personal history of malignant neoplasm of prostate	18
C90.00: Multiple myeloma not having achieved remission	17
C61: Malignant neoplasm of prostate	17
Z85.038: Personal history of other malignant neoplasm of large intestine	16
C78.7: Secondary malignant neoplasm of liver and intrahepatic bile duct	14
C79.51: Secondary malignant neoplasm of bone	13

ICD Cancer Code	Count
C91.10: Chronic lymphocytic leukemia of B-cell type not having achieved remission	12
C91.00: Acute lymphoblastic leukemia not having achieved remission	8
C34.90: Malignant neoplasm of unspecified part of unspecified bronchus or lung	8
C34.11: Malignant neoplasm of upper lobe, right bronchus or lung	8
C78.00: Secondary malignant neoplasm of unspecified lung	8
Z85.118: Personal history of other malignant neoplasm of bronchus and lung	7
C25.9: Malignant neoplasm of pancreas, unspecified	7
C34.91: Malignant neoplasm of unspecified part of right bronchus or lung	7
C34.92: Malignant neoplasm of unspecified part of left bronchus or lung	7
C80.1: Malignant (primary) neoplasm, unspecified	6
C25.0: Malignant neoplasm of head of pancreas	6
J91.0: Malignant pleural effusion	6
C54.1: Malignant neoplasm of endometrium	6
C79.31: Secondary malignant neoplasm of brain	6
C22.8: Malignant neoplasm of liver, primary, unspecified as to type	6
C92.00: Acute myeloblastic leukemia, not having achieved remission	5
C16.9: Malignant neoplasm of stomach, unspecified	5
C18.9: Malignant neoplasm of colon, unspecified	5
C50.912: Malignant neoplasm of unspecified site of left female breast	4
C92.Z0: Other myeloid leukemia not having achieved remission	4
C78.6: Secondary malignant neoplasm of retroperitoneum and peritoneum	4
C85.90: Non-Hodgkin lymphoma, unspecified, unspecified site	4
C54.9: Malignant neoplasm of corpus uteri, unspecified	4
Z85.828: Personal history of other malignant neoplasm of skin	4
C50.919: Malignant neoplasm of unspecified site of unspecified female breast	4
C50.911: Malignant neoplasm of unspecified site of right female breast	4
C23: Malignant neoplasm of gallbladder	4
C78.5: Secondary malignant neoplasm of large intestine and rectum	3
C34.12: Malignant neoplasm of upper lobe, left bronchus or lung	3
Z85.07: Personal history of malignant neoplasm of pancreas	3
C71.9: Malignant neoplasm of brain, unspecified	3
C34.31: Malignant neoplasm of lower lobe, right bronchus or lung	3
C53.9: Malignant neoplasm of cervix uteri, unspecified	3
C78.01: Secondary malignant neoplasm of right lung	3
C20: Malignant neoplasm of rectum	3
C56.9: Malignant neoplasm of unspecified ovary	3

Having identified 480 patients with cancer who had an in-hospital death in 0–180 days before the death admission, we are going to focus the index line on the penultimate discharge so we can calculate the elapsed time between the penultimate discharge and the death hospitalization (Figure 32).

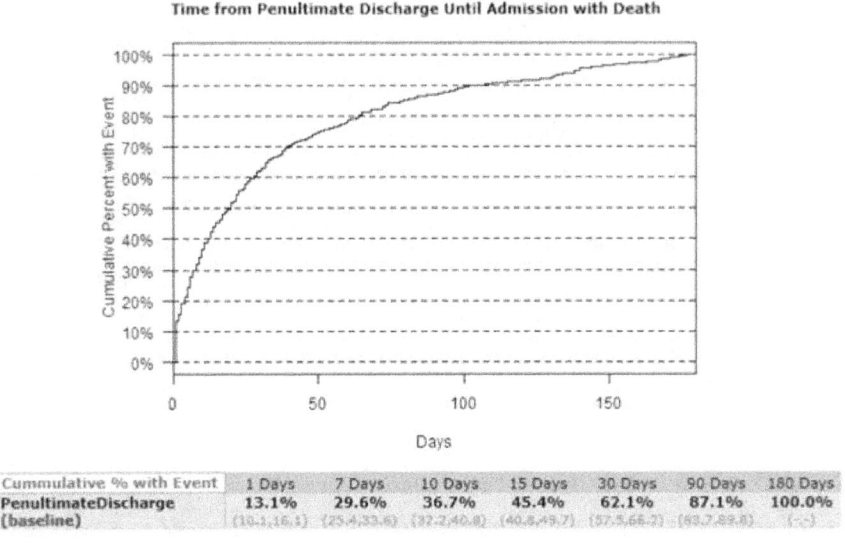

Cummulative % with Event	1 Days	7 Days	10 Days	15 Days	30 Days	90 Days	180 Days
PenultimateDischarge (baseline)	13.1%	29.6%	36.7%	45.4%	62.1%	87.1%	100.0%
	(10.1,16.1)	(25.4,33.6)	(32.2,40.8)	(40.8,49.7)	(57.5,66.2)	(83.7,89.8)	(-,-)

Figure 32. Cumulative incidence admission with death from penultimate hospital discharge

Now find inpatient palliative care consults by adding a condition line requiring the event type "Order Non-Med" using the following palliative care set.

Table 35. Palliative care consult list

Palliative Care Consult
Ped Palliative Care or Pain Consult
IP CONSULT TO PALLIATIVE CARE
AMB REFERRAL TO PALLIATIVE CARE
AMB REFERRAL TO HOME HEALTH PALLIATIVE CARE
IP CONSULT TO PEDIATRIC PALLIATIVE CARE
IP CONSULT TO SPIRITUAL PALLIATIVE CARE
PALLIATIVE CARE ALREADY INVOLVED
EMMI - PALLIATIVE CARE

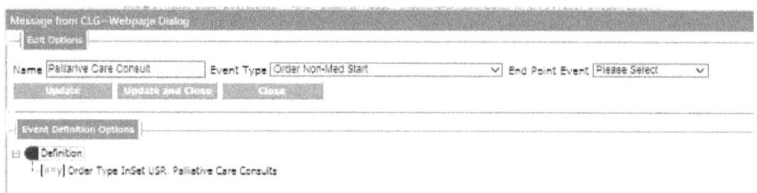

Figure 33. Palliative care consult event (Order Non-Med Start)

Add the fourth condition lines on the event canvas to require a palliative care consult 0–365 days before the index date of the most proximal discharge to the admission of death—the penultimate hospitalization (Figure 34). This query starts at the discharge date of the penultimate hospitalization (the event type is the discharge date with its end point event being the discharge date by default) and looks back 365 days to capture all the inpatient palliative care consults of the penultimate hospitalization as well as any other hospitalization in the antecedent 365 days.

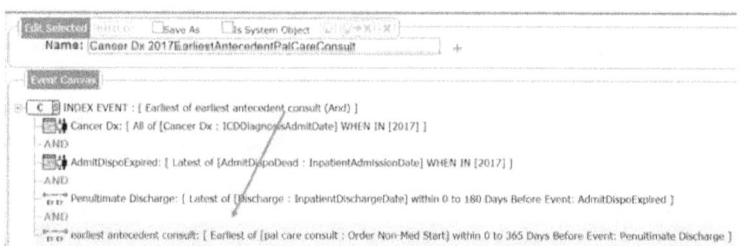

Figure 34. Palliative care consultation 0–365 days before the penultimate discharge (N=211)

211/480 (44%) have a palliative care consultation in the 365 days before the penultimate discharge in 2017.

For those with a palliative care consultation within one year prior to the penultimate discharge, we calculate time elapsed between palliative care consultation and death admission (Figure 35).

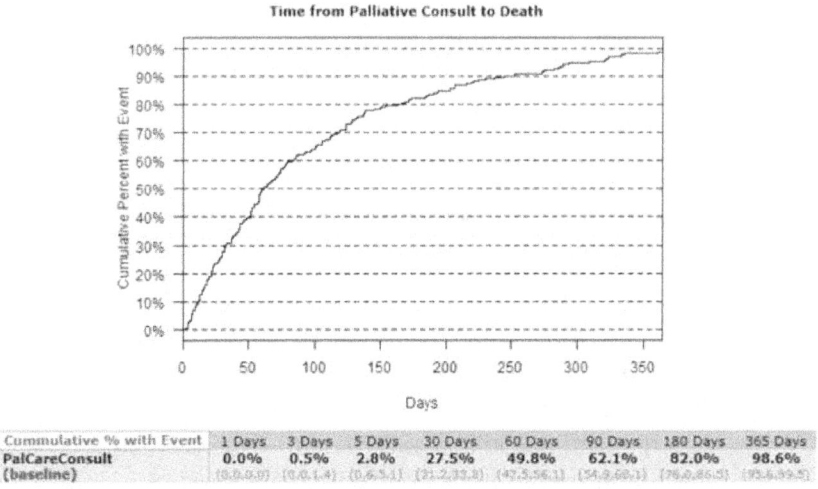

Figure 35. Cumulative incidence palliative consultation until
admission to hospital with disposition=expired in 2017

So 44% of the patients did not have a palliative care consultation at all, and for those 56% who did have a consultation, 62% had the consult 30 days or less prior to the inpatient admission that resulted in death.

Some Considerations

1. Our method required that the patient die in the hospital. Ideally, we would have included death that also occurred outside the hospital, but we do not have this data. Vital Statistic Registries do not provide this information broadly, and Social Security death tapes available to the public are less than 50% complete since 2011.[4] The fact that all our patients died in the hospital may be biased to oversample those patients who did not have palliative consultation. Had they received such consultation, we would have expected that at least some of them would have preferred to die in an in-home hospice or hospice institutions and without a hospital death would have been excluded by our criteria.

2. Palliative care percent as conceived of as wholistic care may be overestimated in our calculations. In conversations with palliative care specialists who also provide pain medication management, I have heard that some

oncologists who do request a consult do so for the pain care management. These oncologists do not cede control of the cadence or extent of the overall care to an outside party and thus limit the scope of palliation to pain medication management instead of wholistic management.

3. Cancer case definition is reliant upon a cancer ICD diagnosis. Alternative case definitions could consider the following:
   a. Tumor Registry
   b. Oncology medication prescribed during inpatient or outpatient treatment to demonstrate active management of the cancer at some point in the year. This choice, while establishing an active engagement with the cancer, would be biased against full ascertainment of patients receiving palliation as those who elected to avoid chemotherapy as part of a palliation plan would be excluded from the calculation.

Predictive Model for Mortality to Guide Palliative Care Consultation: It Is Not the Model but the Will

n another institution I know, a similar problem of inadequate palliative care was recognized. As thoughts turned to a then-new notion of oncologic medical home—a notion of wholistic care for the oncology patient—interest turned toward identifying a priority scheme to provide palliative care consultation. A predictive model was sought to use data available during a hospitalization to predict death in 30 days. With this model in hand, proactive efforts targeting oncology patients not yet in palliative care could enroll those patients to focus on comfort and preclude futile and expensive hospitalization and intensive care unit stay. While no model—no matter how good—could be expected to perfectly predict death, its goal was more limited, and its economic success was justified because consultation is relatively inexpensive compared to hospitalization. Even for a patient incorrectly predicted to die, provision of palliative care consultation would be considered a benefit and ideal standard of care.

Without getting too deep in the weeds, data was collected on the historical behavior of oncology patients with the identification of laboratory tests, medication class, history of medications, Charlson score,[43-46] age and gender, and number of inpatient, outpatient, and emergency room visits in the preceding 180 days. For those patients without the laboratory values, normal values were imputed. Continuous variables were often cut into factor categories as seemed prudent based upon clinical and statistical considerations and maximum and minimum values of variables thought to be important in specific antecedent time windows.

We then followed a conventional statistical process.

1. Partition the data into training and testing subsets of observations (rows).
2. Build the model on the training set.
3. Predict died_in_30 for the testing set.
4. Compare the predicted results with observed results.

The final model was tested by a process of K-fold cross-validation[47] where randomly selected 9/10 of the data was used to build the model and then tested against the held-out portion. The variability in the model's ability to predict death was then attributed to the final model, and it gives a sense of the variability that should be experienced when applying the model to new data.

Our working objective was to produce a model with few false negatives at the cost of tolerating extra false positives. The model was extraordinarily successful (ROC Curve Figure 36) with an extraordinary area under the curve AUC of 0.89.

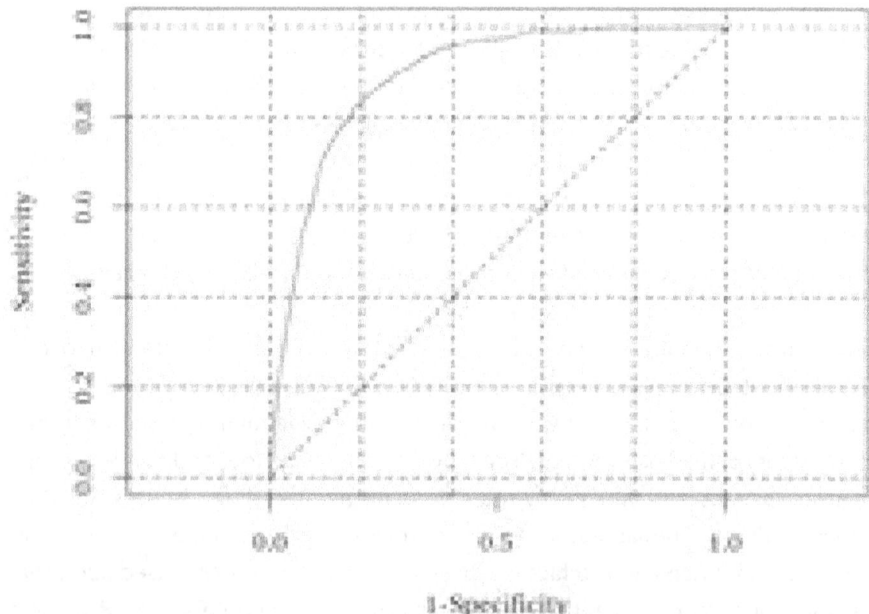

Figure 36. ROC curve for death-predictive analytic (area under curve=.89)

Shown here is a basic 10-fold cross-validation of a test logistic model using a threshold for the indication of death. The mean of the predicted values returned an aggregated contingency table.

Table 36. Results of 10-fold cross-validation

	Observed	
Predicted	Alive	Dead
False	6,417	150
True	1,612	734

This says that out of the 884 (150+734) cases in which death occurred within 30 days of the index event, the model correctly predicts death within 30 days in about 83% (734/884). However, the model also yields false positives in 20% (1,612/8,029 cases).

The real-world performance of the health care system in question without the benefit of the predictive model provided palliative care consultation in only 37% of the cases prior to death. Thus, the predictive model would have improved performance from 37% to 83% but would have tolerated 1,612 false positives.

The model with a positive predictive value of 30% would have had you provide palliative care consultation for 3.2 people in order to capture one true positive.

This is a reasonable tradeoff given the expectation that early palliative care consultation should be a goal of cancer care, anyway.

The postscript is actually the most interesting part of the story. After demonstrating the potential of this model, the institution elected not to implement it. The explanation was this: "We have decided to give palliative care consultations to every cancer patient." To date, this has not occurred.

I suspect that patient ownership disagreement between oncologists and palliative care consultants with oncologists controlling the referral was the cause.

You can build the best models, but if there is no will, there is no way.

Chaos Begets Chaos but Is Reversible with Accountability

―――

earning health systems encourage individuals to evaluate episodes of care to detect unnecessary waste and remediable poor performance. A sequence of profound waste will be described to make this clear. A group of clinicians noticed a 12-week delay to obtain pediatric MRIs. Pediatric anesthesiologists are a scarce resource, and the pediatric MRI requires coordination between pediatric anesthesiologists as well as radiologists because young children need to be anesthetized to obtain a good image. A careful review of the fishbone identified multiple contributors to inefficiency.

1. The patient's family did not know where they should park.
2. The patient's family did not know where to go when they arrived at the hospital for their procedure.
3. Upon arrival to the MRI,
   a. the admission staff needed to record the patient's arrival,
   b. the nurses needed to review care procedures and review history,
   c. the pediatric anesthesiologist needed to be paged and begin their procedure, and
   d. the radiology tech needed to activate the MRI.

All of these steps were compromised with delays. With each corruption, downstream clinical actors saw that being on time served no purpose, and their other responsibilities began taking priority, further delaying the first-procedure start time so that the start was delayed by an average of an hour and a half.

Tightening up each of these steps—first with parking assistance, then with clear directions for patients, and then followed by tight surveillance of the clinical actors with immediate accountability—converted supervisory indifference and provider sloth to a tight patient flow with clinicians on site on time. The net result was that scheduling latency reduced from 12 weeks to 12 days without hiring additional staff.

The important lesson here is that systems and their internal components adapt to expectations and harvest chaos when performance expectations are not diligently and consistently enforced.

Temporally Boutique Improvement: Projects without Sustainability

A serious failure of some health systems that express interest in performance improvement is that they have learned how to engage in episodic evaluation and remediation, even encouraging participation of their training house staff with dramatic results, but they make no provision for sustainability. This need for an institutional vision to create the infrastructure to easily convert transient success to permanent success will be explicitly described in the next example.

Surgical procedures sometimes require Kefzol antibiotic prophylaxis to prevent infection. However, the pharmacokinetics requires redosing with the same dose as the initial one if the surgery duration is longer than four hours. Unfortunately, three errors are prevalent: failure to initially dose, failure to redose if surgery duration is prolonged, and failure to redose with the adequate dose. Correcting the initial failure-to-dose error can be achieved by using a checklist, but redosing and appropriate dosing by the anesthesiologist requires a computer alert as well as clinician education.

Evaluating the effect of the alert required a manual review of the surgeries for which Kefzol was prescribed and for which the duration was longer than four hours. This manual review to identify the relevant patients was then evaluated by a manual review for the fact of repeat dosing as well as the dose of that second infusion.

The improvement effort demonstrated a dramatic increase in appropriate second dosing, an impressive success. However, to sustain this success, we must have automated surveillance not dependent on the zeal of residents who heroically performed the manual review. We need in our data warehouse the start and end time of operations and the medication dose and time.

But this is just one project. A visionary institution creates a warehouse that provides core data events, time, and values, plus reusable temporal analytic patterns to support both ad hoc and routine surveillance[3,4] so that when new projects such as these demonstrate effectiveness, they can be rapidly converted into ongoing surveillance.

Failure of Temporal Alignment

The rapid dissolution of clots in affected cerebral vessels is critical to saving a stroke victim from permanent disability. Even with relatively rapid intervention, under optimal conditions, our ability to achieve patient functionality, which is defined minimally as walking with the aid of a walker at 90 days instead of being paralyzed, can be achieved with our present technology 30% of the time. Critical to success is the rapidity with which a radiologic diagnosis can be made and therapy initiated.

Our organization tracks the elapsed time from the patient presentation to the emergency room door until the intra-arterial infusion of a clot-busting agent. A graph of our success at a timely infusion is shown as the average time per quarter (lower is better).

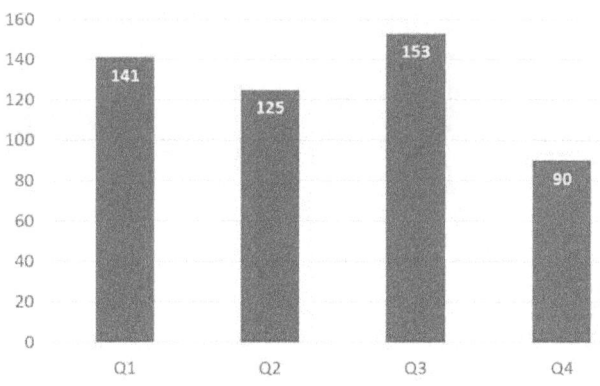

Figure 37. Average minutes to reperfusion by quarter

A graph of outcomes is provided below (higher is better). Each month, we interview people on the 90th day after the infusion, and we provide the percent who have meaningful function below.

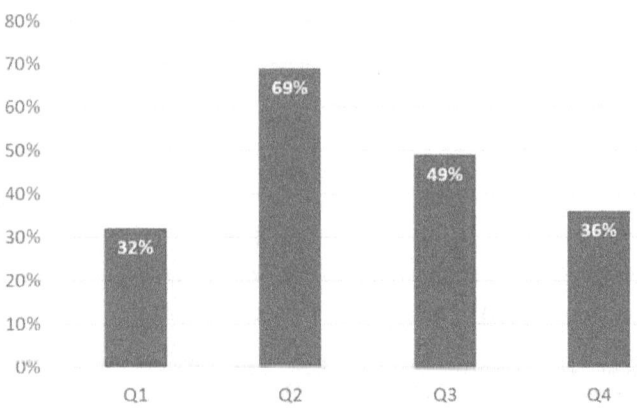

Independent at 90 days 2018

Figure 38. Functional independence at 90 days by quarter in 2018

What do you notice?

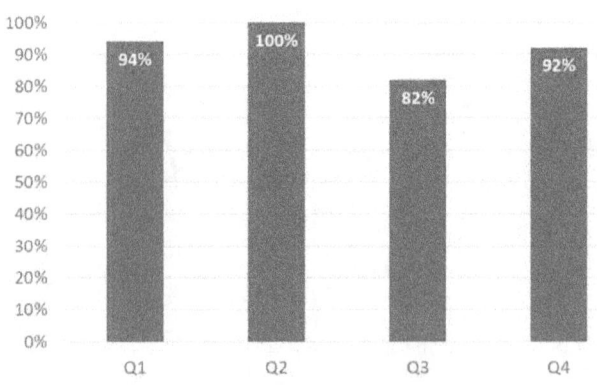

Successful reperfusion 2018

Figure 39. Percent successful reperfusion by quarter in 2018

While there is a dramatic reduction in the time until infusion, we are not seeing improvement in functionality (Figure 38). Why?

1. Is it possible that there is some time threshold that must be achieved to see an improvement? Dropping to 90 minutes on average may not be low enough to actually result in an observable improvement.
2. The key metric is not being properly represented with temporal alignment of the appropriate exposure with its outcome. Remember that when you are looking at time to infusion and outcome, you must make sure that both are referring to the same cohort. If you are looking at a stroke cohort from January 2019, summarizing its average time until the clot-buster infusion, you must associate this exposure with the outcome measure observed 90 days later in April 2019. The present graphic incorrectly assigns the outcome to the date of the outcome interview, not to the date of the exposed cohort.

Interestingly enough, there is another challenge that will soon impact our graphical success. In fact, it will be our very successes that will drive a worsening of our metrics unless we approach the metric with a degree of insight and subtlety.

As Montefiore's reputation for excellence in stroke intervention grows, more patients will be referred to Montefiore from other emergency rooms for clot busting. We should expect worsening of our reported outcomes as a result. Why?

The metric we are now using measures elapsed time from presentation to the Montefiore emergency room to medication infusion. As a first-generation metric, it is reasonable. We want to optimize those processes completely under our control within the walls of our hospital. However, the biologically relevant elapsed time is the time from the clot manifestation in the patient's home until the time of the clot dissolution in the hospital. When receiving patients from another facility, the relevant elapsed time is not the time from the Montefiore emergency room door but rather the time from the stroke onset at home until the medication infusion. Patients referred from another emergency room experience additional delays in transportation and diagnosis even before they reach our hospital entrance.

To address this concern in our reporting, we ought to separate the patients first presenting to Montefiore from those presenting elsewhere and capture the time from that elsewhere to the clot-busting infusion with careful attention to transportation and diagnosis delays. System-wide resources must be planned and organized to reduce this additional time in which the clot is undissolved.

As our reputation attracts additional stroke patients, our emergency room will be challenged by additional high-criticality patients whose care trumps that of all others, further delaying processing of those already in our emergency room. In addition, for those who rule out for a remediable clot, these nonclot patients with acute neurologic findings will add to our overload both in the emergency room and in their subsequent hospitalization. This is something for which we must plan.

Error-Proofing Clinical Care: Build Learning in Structure

A case was reviewed that related the following. A patient had a deep wound that was emergently packed with multiple pledgets. A number of days later, a different house officer surgeon removed the pledgets and closed the wound. A few days later, the wound began to suppurate, and when the wound was reopened, retained pledgets were discovered.

Discussion turned to the issue of the cause of the error. Some focused on the fact that the original surgical house staff was not the house staff member who removed the pledgets. Implicit in this comment was the mistaken belief that the same house staff member would retain the count memory over three days. Others suggested that the surgical procedure note should have included the number of pledgets. But this, too, is subject to counting errors as well as sloppiness in performance. The last suggestion involved the realization that individual pledgets are, by their very nature, an accident waiting to happen. House staff should be required to use continuous gauze so that once you start to pull out the gauze, there is physical continuity of the rest of the gauze, making it impossible to leave any behind.

The latter approach is a method of baking in the knowledge of the first error in a force function that precludes its repetition. This is the sort of low-tech-embedded learning that survives forever.

The Academic Nanite as Agent of Change

The learning health system needs easy access to raw data as well as to software with reusable temporal patterns[3,7] that can support spontaneous exploration without the need for the services of a technical priesthood. Since the number of potential questions are infinite and available analysts are always finite, academic medical centers need to take advantage of their large training force (residents, fellows, faculty) to evaluate the process of care and ask novel questions.

These agents are academic nanites swarming over the institution's information space to ferret out failures or opportunities for improvement. They ought to see themselves as members of an integrated delivery system where patient need trumps fealty to siloed departmental interests. They must provide critical, timely feedback to clinical partners in different sites as we have discussed in the example of the emergency department providing timely follow-up to the outpatient clinics when they encounter an unnecessary emergency department visit. This feedback loop provides the data that their clinic partners cannot produce on their own to inform their continuous improvement processes.

This approach enriches the training experience of the trainees and sharpens the thought processes of the faculty. With each search of the database data flow defects can be identified and repaired to the benefit of all.

The described infrastructure reality is a marked deviation from the standard grant-funded activity that fuels research in most institutions by hiring a highly specialized data extractor to pull out a dataset that is then fully cleaned and curated by the researcher. The individual federally funded exercise leaves nothing useful behind to sustain surveillance or enable additional analyses. This wasteful cycle ignores the principle of sustainability or scalability. Unfortunately, the academic enterprise is built upon this model and is self-reinforcing.

Learning Health System as Witness to and Watchdog of Federal Policy Error

Among its useful social functions, the learning health system can bear witness to the consequences of implemented federal policy serving as a check on policy errors. In 2008, Segal et al.[48] did just that—evaluating the impact of the strict enforcement of an old rule ignored in practice since 1983. The rule, called the 75 percent rule at the time, threatened inpatient rehabilitation facilities with the loss of their Medicare eligibility status if the percent of patients in their facility with appropriate diagnoses fell below 75 percent. This economic threat resulted in a dramatic change in referral patterns from acute care hospitals who, before the enforcement, relied upon clinical determinations based upon medical and psychosocial factors.

Hospital efforts to reduce length of stay resulted in the discharge of patients in a feebler state than was heretofore the norm requiring additional rehabilitation. The federal economic drivers pressured both the hospitals to discharge early and the nursing homes to reject admissions, creating a growing cohort of patients who were consigned to a zone of neglect purgatory.

I should be clear that federal policy is implemented without an expectation of evaluation, so the frailest members of our society were subjected to an in vivo experiment without anyone required to evaluate the consequences.

Fortunately, a resident in rehabilitation medicine used Clinical Looking Glass to build cohorts of patients aged 65 or older, discharged with the diagnoses proscribed by the 75 percent rule, before and after the rule's enforcement. The results were striking. There was an increase in readmissions greatest for pain syndromes (from 33 to 55 percent) and in patients older than 85 with orthopedic diagnoses, and the mortality rate increased from 25 to 54 percent. Cardiac and pulmonary patients died more frequently and were more likely to be readmitted after strict enforcement.

Backstory

A physical medicine and rehabilitation (PM&R) resident was a second-year resident in her third trimester of pregnancy going to Greece for a vacation when her 80-year-old grandmother, who had been previously fully ambulatory without a cane or walker and living on her own, suffered an acute thrombotic ischemic occlusion of her leg. Prior to leaving for vacation, the resident instructed her family to make sure that her grandma was sent to acute rehabilitation. She explicitly warned the family to ignore any doctor or social worker who advised referral to a nursing home. However, upon return from her long-overdue vacation, the resident found her grandmother lying in a nursing home bed, infected with a multidrug-resistant urinary tract infection, and at the head of the bed she saw a sign declaring that her grandma was demented. With great effort, the resident eventually got her grandmother transferred to an active rehabilitation facility. Her grandma subsequently recovered enough to return to fully independent living with an excellent quality of life for an additional six years. She died at home.

The resident was infuriated and wanted to prevent this from recurring. She recognized that the 75 percent rule was the ultimate culprit, denying those who were debilitated but without the correct diagnosis needed rehabilitation. This rule was especially a problem for small facilities that could not tolerate accepting incorrect-diagnosis patients because they did not have enough volume of the right patient types to dilute out the wrong ones and protect them from federal punishment should an audit occur.

She wanted to get the word out but was advised to write a case report. Unhappy with this suggestion, she planned with a colleague to devise some sort of study, and they put together the elements for the Institutional Review Board application. It was there, when she spoke of her need to get access to data, that she was informed about the existence of Clinical Looking Glass (CLG). She met with me and was trained.

Fortunately, the American Hospital Association had previously put together a list of the diagnoses for which a rehabilitation referral was permitted as well as a list of those that were ineligible. Furthermore, because there was a period of rule suspension and a period of rule enforcement, cohorts could be built to test the impact of the rule implementation. Once the cohorts were built and the effect was demonstrated, additional institutional support was provided for statistical help, resulting in the write-up and publication. The resident chose to stay at Montefiore as an attending for a year post training to complete the analysis and write-up.

Ultimately, the paper was published in the *PM&R* and was cited in the American Academy of Physical Medicine and Rehabilitation as the best paper of the year, and the physician served for two three-year terms as a member of the academy's health care policy committee.

The nursing home "right diagnosis threshold" is, at the time of this writing, set at 60 percent. I am told that many smaller programs have closed because they have not been able to withstand this requirement. The rule worsens disparity as only those with advocates or wealth can overcome the inherent disincentive created by the 60 percent diagnosis-restrictive rule.

Debilitated elderly are the prey of this rule and subject to zombie reactivation of its implementation as pressure for CMS savings recur and memories of the impact fade. It is the transparency enabled by CLG and the heart of engaged clinicians that man the wall against the zombie hordes of bad policies with impacts that, while they are otherwise invisible, cause needless suffering and magnify inequities.

Learning Health System as Witness to Opiate Prescription Intervention Success

n the first two decades of the 21st century, the United States suffered from an epidemic of premature death due to opiate overdose with prescription medications involved in 36 to 42 percent of cases.[49,50] Medical culture in the preceding two decades in the previous century had loosened attitudes toward the use of narcotics emphasizing pain control in nononcologic settings and building expectations of a pain-free existence by treating pain as the fifth vital sign. Because it was considered the fifth vital sign, this meant that it deserved the same attention and response due to blood pressure, pulse, respiratory rate, or temperature.

Some suspect that part of the national addiction problem was created through the liberal use of narcotics with the resultant iatrogenic addiction of the population. Of course, there were other powerful economic drivers in the pharmaceutical distribution chain that are only now undergoing scrutiny, but we will focus on the potential role of the medical system and its ability to monitor its response to the challenge.

If we believe that unnecessarily prescribed narcotics contributed to the opiate epidemic and that new policies have since reduced the medical community's contribution to this plague, how would you design a metric to monitor the success of remediation efforts?

The exposure of a narcotic to a narcotic-naïve patient by the medical care system is the starting point. There are three loci of exposure: inpatient hospitalization, the emergency department, and the outpatient clinic visit. For a first-order evaluation of an unnecessary opioid prescription, you would want to eliminate cancer patients to eliminate patients with an obvious clinical justification and whose survival horizon is constrained. Of course, there can be inappropriate use of narcotics in early-stage pain-free disease, but we are trying to build a crude first metric.

Now we need a metric to meaningfully demonstrate chronic population dependence. For this quick and dirty exercise, we will consider a repeat narcotic prescription in days 365–730 after the index date of first exposure. This outcome measure is, in a sense, a summary measure of all the attitudes and influences of the entire learning health care system in its multiple interactions with the patient over time to sustain the use of the narcotic. Every subsequent outpatient, emergency department, or inpatient prescription will reinforce, sustain, attenuate, or eliminate this behavior. In a sense, the single measure one to two years after the first exposure is somewhat akin to a HgbA1c integrating the blood glucose level experience of the patient over time. If the learning health system is encouraging dependence, then we would expect from a population perspective that this percent prescription persistence metric to increase. Admittedly, this is a crude analysis, but it gives you an approach to obtain a global understanding of a multifactorial and multicomponent process effect.

Using Clinical Looking Glass, we will examine groups of initially oxycodone- (or opiate-) naïve patients in the Montefiore inpatient, emergency department, or outpatient settings to answer the question, "Has our practice of medicine over secular time worsened oxycodone or opiate dependence?"

While we cannot establish causality with any certainty, we can at least describe secular trends in persistent outpatient use of oxycodone (or opiates) after the first introduction in the inpatient, emergency room, or outpatient setting. Persistent use will be defined as evidence of at least one prescription of oxycodone 365–730 days after first exposure in any of the three Montefiore sites.

Create cohorts based upon first use of oxycodone in oxycodone-naïve patients in the years 2016, 2013, 2010, and 2007. Oxycodone will be any medication containing oxycodone. The set used is provided in Table 37.

Table 37. Oxycodone medication

Assigned list
ibuprofen/oxycodone HCl
oxycodone HCl
oxycodone HCl,terephth/aspirin
oxycodone HCl/acetaminophen
oxycodone HCl/aspirin
oxycodone HCl/naltrexone HCl
oxycodone myristate
oxycodone/aspirin

To demonstrate our method, we will work through inpatient 2016 considerations. This inpatient admission has three exclusions:

1. The patient could not have received oxycodone as an in-hospital medication at any time in the past 1–3650 days (10 years) before hospital admission—event type "Med Order Start."
2. The patient could not have received oxycodone as an outpatient medication at any time in the past 1–3650 days (10 years) before hospital admission—event type "Prescription Written."
3. The patient did not have cancer documented in the Montefiore Tumor Registry in the prior 1–3650 days before the visit—event type "Cancer Registry—Initial."

To find the year 2016 inpatient oxycodone-naïve cohort prior to hospitalization without evidence of cancer, we build the following four condition lines in Clinical Looking Glass and identify 42,232 patients (Figure 40).

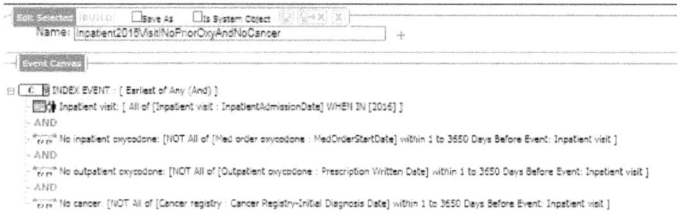

Figure 40. Oxycodone-naïve hospitalized patients (counted only once if hospitalized more than once) without evidence of cancer (N=42,232)

We now want to identify which of these oxycodone-naïve patients were given oxycodone during their inpatient stay. We accomplish this by adding an additional condition line "oxycodone during admission" (Figure 41) that demands a new event, Med Order (medication set=oxycodone), occurring during the inpatient visit by using the "when in" durational temporal operator pointing to the admission condition line. The oxycodone medication order occurred during the inpatient hospitalization.

These are oxycodone naifs receiving oxycodone for the first time ever during their 2016 hospitalization (N=8,199).

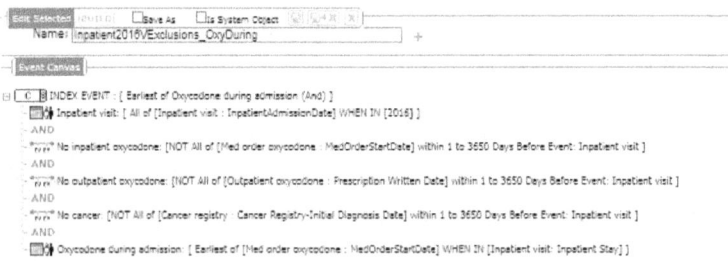

Figure 41. Oxycodone-naïve hospitalized patient without evidence of cancer prescribed oxycodone for the first time (N=8,199)

"Naif" may be a bit of an overstatement, as we only have information from our own medical system and cannot state with certainty that the patient never received these medications from another system.

To identify those potentially addicted by this first in-hospital exposure followed by an ongoing health system relationship, we will find those who had an outpatient prescription for oxycodone within 365–730 days after the first in-hospital oxycodone administration without a cancer diagnosis (Figure 42).

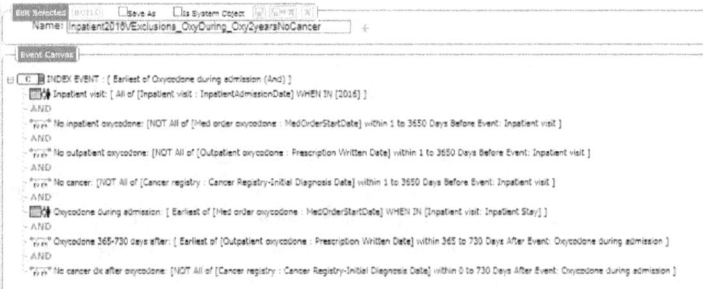

Figure 42. Persistent oxycodone prescription 365–730 days post first exposure as an inpatient (N=507)

Out of the total 8,199 oxycodone naifs, 507 or 6.2% of individuals were prescribed oxycodone within 365–730 days after their first exposure without any evidence of cancer within two years of their original oxycodone exposure.

Repeating the process for 2016, 2013, 2010, and 2007 yields Table 38.

Table 38. Persistence of oxycodone use after first-time inpatient exposure

Inpatient Oxycodone							
	2016	2015	2014	2013	2011	2010	2007
Oxycodone-naïve hospitalized patient (counted only once if multiply hospitalized) without evidence of cancer	42,232	43,145	43,721	43,672	44,271	46,479	38,905
Oxycodone naïve hospitalized patient without evidence of cancer-prescribed oxycodone for the first time	8,199	8,951	9,444	9,533	6,995	7,701	8,579
Patients with persistent oxycodone outpatient prescriptions 365–730 days after initial exposure and no evidence of cancer two years post prescription	507	672	826	924	799	817	901
Percent of patients with persistent oxycodone use	6.2	7.5	8.7	9.7	11.4	10.6	10.5

We note a clear downward trend of persistent prescriptions percent, suggesting that our efforts to contain dependence is improving. Keep in mind that patients exposed in 2016 are being evaluated by the presence of an oxycodone prescription in 2018.

A simple logistic model looking at year as a factor (baseline 2007), neighborhood socioeconomic status,[12] gender (baseline female), and age at first exposure yields the following (Table 39).

Table 39. Logistic regression model persistent prescription after inpatient exposure

		Confidence	Interval
	Odds Ratios	2.5%	97.5%
Intercept	.099	.088	.11

Age at Exposure	.996	.994	.997
GenderM	1.05	.98	1.12
SocioEconomicStatus	.96	.95	.97
Year Factor2010*	1.09	.97	1.21
YearFactor2011	1.19	1.07	1.33
YearFactor2013	.97	.88	1.08
YearFactor2014	.87	.78	.97
YearFactor2015	.75	.67	.84
YearFactor2016	.62	.54	.70

*base year 2007

Now we will study the outpatient setting.

We can do this in Looking Glass easily by modifying existing work. Change the event type in the first condition line from inpatient admission to outpatient visit (Figure 43).

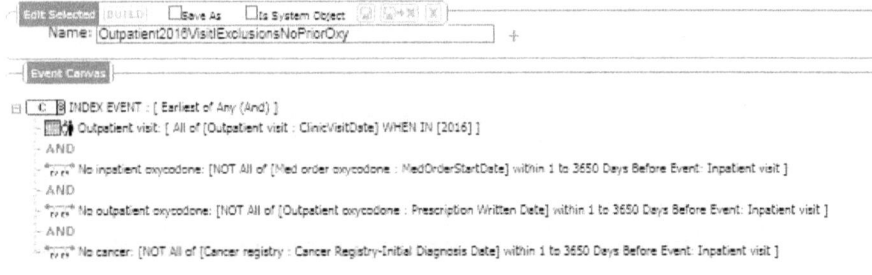

Figure 43. Oxycodone-naïve outpatients in 2016 without a diagnosis of cancer (N=390,381)

This yields 390,381 outpatient oxycodone naifs without oxycodone exposure or Tumor Registry evidence of cancer prior to a Montefiore outpatient visit in 2016.

We will now look for an oxycodone prescription given within 0–24 hours around (before or after) the date of the outpatient visit (Figure 44).

Important note: In our information system, outpatient visit date:time was set to midnight before our latest EMR (Epic) implementation. Because of this, we need to look 0–24 hours around the date of the visit to find a medication prescription associated with the outpatient visit. After the Epic implementation, we have the exact date:time of the outpatient visit, but to maintain consistency of the analysis across time, we must use the less precise approach forced upon us by the earlier data.

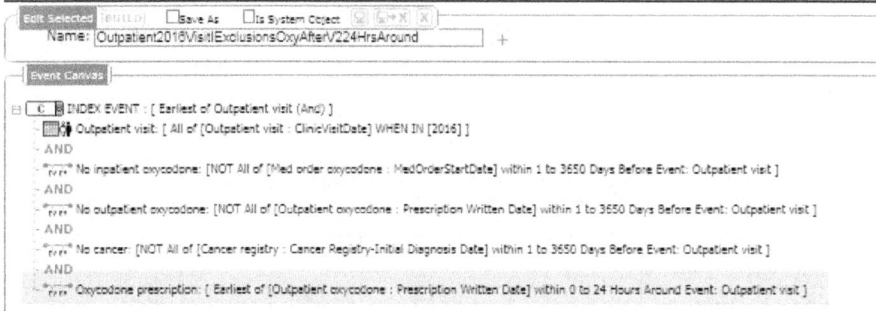

Figure 44. Oxycodone-naïve outpatients in 2016 without a cancer
diagnosis prescribed oxycodone (N=2,566)

2,566 oxycodone-naïve outpatients without cancer prior to the outpatient visit received an oxycodone prescription in the outpatient setting in 2016.

Now we seek those given another prescription for oxycodone 365–730 days after the first exposure (condition line 7, Figure 45). We will also require the absence of Tumor Registry evidence of cancer in the 2 years post initial oxycodone exposure.

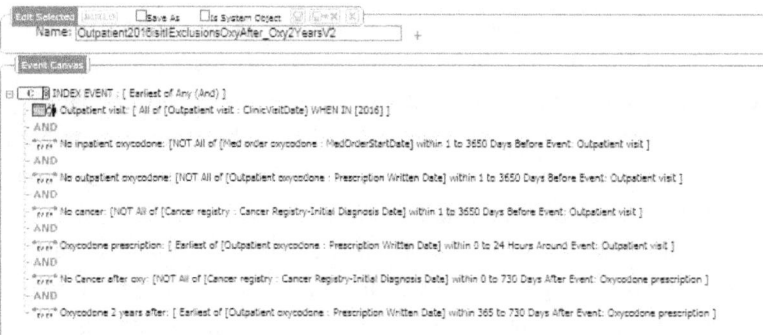

Figure 45. Oxycodone-naïve outpatients in 2016 without a cancer diagnosis prescribed
oxycodone with persistent prescription 365–730 days after (N=248)

248 people had another oxycodone prescription 365–730 days after the first prescription.

Repeat the process for 2016, 2013, 2010, and 2007 (Table 40).

Table 40. Persistent oxycodone use in oxycodone-naïve outpatients in 2016 without a cancer diagnosis prescribed oxycodone

Outpatient Oxycodone							
	2016	2015	2014	2013	2011	2010	2007
Oxycodone-naïve Outpatient (counted only once) without evidence of cancer	390,381	377,110	375,976	368,378	353,608	350,264	251,025
Oxycodone naïve Outpatient without evidence of cancer-prescribed oxycodone	2,566	5,500	5,088	4,601	3,780	3,016	1,305
Patients with persistent oxycodone outpatient prescriptions 365–730 days after initial exposure and no evidence of cancer two years post prescription	248	478	599	636	791	622	693
Percent of patients with persistent oxycodone use	9.7	8.7	11.8	13.8	20.9	20.6	53.1

We note again that oxycodone percent persistence drops from 2010 through 2015 with a surprising increase in 2016. The percent increases but not the absolute number because the number exposed to oxycodone dropped dramatically from 5,500 to 2,566. Perhaps the percent increase is due to the more appropriate reduction of first exposure to those who really ought to have the treatment initially and who legitimately should have persistence.

We see a very low outpatient oxycodone exposure in 2007 and might therefore suspect that there might a sensitivity problem to outpatient prescription of any sort, not just oxycodone in 2007. We search for any medication order associated with cohort members and look for secular trends (Table 41).

Table 41. EMR outpatient sensitivity for prescriptions

Outpatient Oxycodone				
	2016	2013	2010	2007
Outpatient oxycodone naifs without prior evidence of cancer	390,381	368,378	350,264	251,025

Outpatient oxycodone naifs without prior evidence of cancer prescribed any medication	212,993	235,660	201,001	175,857
Percent of patients with a prescription of any medication	55	64	57	70

Although there are fewer prescriptions in 2007, a consequence of a smaller health care system at the time, the percent of patients with at least one prescription is, if anything, greater in 2007. This suggests that we do not have evidence of a lack of sensitivity to outpatient prescription. The variability in prescriptions is unexplained.

Next, we will look at oxycodone in the emergency department for patients whose disposition was discharged to home. The data shows the following.

Table 42. Persistence of oxycodone prescription for oxycodone-naïve patients first exposed to oxycodone in ED

Emergency Department Oxycodone							
	2016	2015	2014	2013	2011	2010	2007
Oxycodone-naïve emergency department patients without evidence of cancer	126,887	131,038	129,048	124,791	121,015	122,041	98,498
Oxycodone-naïve emergency department patients without evidence of cancer prescribed oxycodone	8,053	10,243	9,925	9,002	6,947	7,497	5,051
Patients with persistent oxycodone outpatient prescriptions 365–730 days after initial exposure and no evidence of cancer two years post prescription	383	642	718	783	728	876	639
% of patients with persistent oxycodone use	4.8	6.3	7.2	8.7	10.5	11.7	12.7

Next, look at the entire class of opiates, not just oxycodone alone.

Table 43. Opiate persistence after first exposure as inpatients

Inpatient Opiates							
	2016	2015	2014	2013	2011	2010	2007
Opiate-naïve hospitalized patients without evidence of cancer	35,480	36,272	36,862	36,770	37,753	39,870	33,522
Opiate-naïve hospitalized patients without evidence of cancer-prescribed opiate	13,690	11,810	12,503	12535	9,542	10,308	10,806
Patients with persistent opiate outpatient prescriptions 365–730 days after initial exposure and no evidence of cancer two years post prescription	1,828	1,979	2,443	2,671	2,577	2,601	2,172
Percentage of patients with persistent opiate use	13.4	16.8	19.5	21.3	27.0	25.2	20.1

Table 44. Opiate persistence after first exposure in emergency department

Emergency Department Opiates							
	2016	2015	2014	2013	2011	2010	2007
Opiate-naïve emergency department patient without evidence of cancer	110,519	113,887	112,152	108,236	105,663	106,988	88,015
Opiate-naïve emergency department patient without evidence of cancer- prescribed opiate	10,378	12,557	11,899	10,811	7,416	8,367	9,935

| Patients with persistent opiate outpatient prescriptions 365–730 days after initial exposure and no evidence of cancer two years post prescription | 549 | 819 | 975 | 1,017 | 873 | 1,136 | 1,473 |
| Percentage of patients with persistent opiate use | 5.3 | 6.5 | 8.2 | 9.4 | 11.8 | 13.6 | 14.8 |

Outpatient Opiates

Table 45. Opiate persistence after first exposure in the outpatient

Outpatient Opiates							
	2016	**2015**	**2014**	**2013**	**2011**	**2010**	**2007**
Opiate-naïve outpatient without evidence of cancer	350,236	334,827	331,929	324,590	314,909	313,970	232,585
Opiate-naïve outpatient without evidence of cancer-prescribed opiate	4,032	7,733	8,033	8,958	8,872	7,700	4,811
Patients with persistent opiate outpatient prescriptions 365–730 days after initial exposure and no evidence of cancer two years post prescription	522	783	1,146	1,626	2,171	2,001	1,541
Percentage of patients with persistent opiate use	12.9	10.1	14.3	18.2	24.5	26.0	32.0

In Table 45, we note a consistent decline of percent persistence opiates over time with the same increase in the outpatient group between 2015 and 2016 seen and explained in the oxycodone outpatient analysis.

Our metric results support the notion that our learning health system has implemented policies and procedures that have reduced the prevalence of prescription-induced dependence. Among those are the New York State emergency room restrictions of opiate prescriptions to five days and the Greater New York Hospital Association initiative restricting this even further to three days and to the use of short-acting opiates. The attention of the press has been of great benefit in creating an atmosphere and expectation between patients and providers, so providers are more hesitant to prescribe opiates than they used to be. E-prescribing, and its additional time-consuming steps when prescribing controlled substances, further discourage their use.

I-STOP/PMP: Internet System for Tracking Overprescribing

The Prescription Monitoring Program,[51] effective August 27, 2013, required most prescribers to consult the Prescription Monitoring Program (PMP) Registry when writing prescriptions for Schedule II, III, and IV controlled substances. The PMP Registry provided practitioners with direct, secure access to view dispensed controlled substance prescription histories for their patients. The PMP is available 24 hours a day, 7 days a week, via an application on the Health Commerce System (HCS) at https://commerce.health.state.ny.us. Patient reports include all controlled substances that were dispensed in New York State and reported by the pharmacy or dispenser for the past year.

For any system perturbation, a broader perspective than a single metric is required. Just because you have successfully reduced the represcription of opiates in individuals initially naïve to opioids does not mean that you have necessarily reversed the opiate addiction-fueled overdose problem. Those who were addicted but not able to obtain prescription sources may turn to illicit drugs to feed their hunger, replacing prescription overdoses with illegal heroin and fentanyl overdoses.

Hospital Revenue and Diagnoses at End of Life for Those Who Die in Hospital: Suggestion for Intervention

The learning health system becomes acutely aware of costs when it enters into capitated relationships with payors. In such relationships, the LHS receives a fixed monthly payment for a group of patients out of which all their clinical expenses must be paid. Suddenly, revenue becomes cost. To give the reader a sense of the extent of this cost, we look at hospital revenue for the patients who died in our three Bronx hospitals in 2017. Of course, we are unable to account for visits to other hospitals, but the results even in a single system are large enough to draw attention.

For the analysis, we will use hospital-collected revenue as proxy for cost in the one week (seven days), one month (30 days), six months (180 days), and a year (365 days) before the date of death, including the cost of the terminal hospitalization.

First, build a cohort of patients who were discharged from the hospital in 2017 and died in the hospital using disposition=expired.

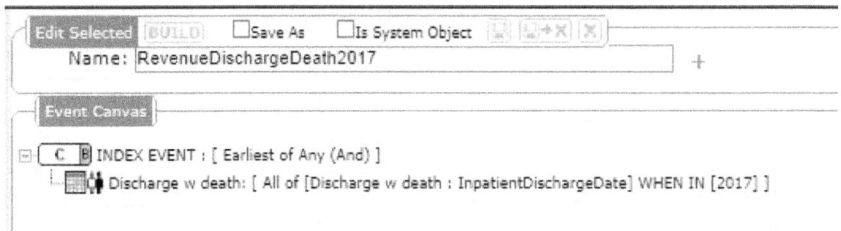

Figure 46. Inpatient cohort who died in hospital in 2017

There were 1,994 patients discharged in 2017 who died during their hospitalization.

Bring the cohort into Study Designer and create a separate analysis definition looking for revenue costs in the preceding 7, 30, 180, and 365 days prior to the patient's death while hospitalized.

This is an example of an analysis definition.

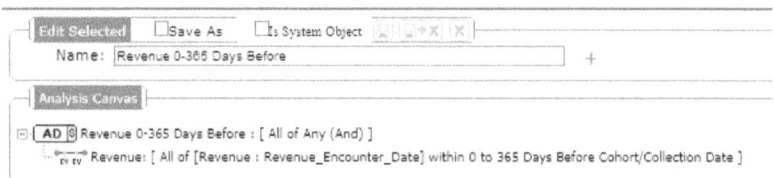

Figure 47. Revenue analysis definition capturing 365 days of inpatient revenue

Running the revenue analysis yields the following.

Table 46. Hospital revenue inclusive of terminal hospitalization by interval

Interval Total Dollars		Cost per person (n=1994)
0–7 Days	$100,817,685.83	$50,815.37
0–30 Days	$113,515,842.14	$57,215.65
0–180 Days	$160,279,904.32	$80,786.24
0–365 Days	$185,452,447.22	$93,474.02

Table 47. Count of patients by revenue interval 0–365 days before death

Revenue (dollars)	Count	Percent
0–25,000	423	21.21
25,000–50,000	394	19.76
50,000–75,000	348	17.45
75,000–100,000	223	11.18
100,000–150,000	227	11.38
150,000–200,000	140	7.02
200,000–300,000	109	5.47
≥300,000	87	4.36
Missing	43	2.16

Table 48. Count of patients by revenue interval 0–7 days before death

Revenue (dollars)	Count	Percent
0–25,000	911	45.64
25,000–50,000	332	16.63
50,000–75,000	380	19.04
75,000–100,000	78	3.91
100,000–150,000	52	2.61
150,000–200,000	58	2.91
200,000–300,000	44	2.2
≥300,000	30	1.5
Missing	111	5.56

Find APR DRG for those patients who died during a hospitalization in 2017.

Table 49. APR DRG for discharges with in-hospital death in 2017

	Count	Cumulative PCT
Septicemia & Disseminated Infections	397	21%
Infect/Parasitic Diseases Inc HIV W OR Proc	262	35%
Moderately Extensive Proc Unrelat To Princ Dx	111	40%
Trach W Long Term Mech Vent W Ext Procedure	86	45%
Heart Failure	84	49%
Other Vascular Procedures	43	52%
CVA & Precerebral Occlusion w/ Infarct	41	54%
Intracranial Hemorrhage	37	56%
Respiratory Malignancy	34	57%
Digestive Malignancy	32	59%
Oth Hepatobiliary, Pancreas & Abdominal Proc	28	61%
Renal Failure	26	62%
Acute Myocardial Infarction	23	63%
Pulmonary Edema & Respiratory Failure	21	64%
Oth OR Proc for Lymph/Hematopoietic/Oth Neopl	21	65%

Malignancy of Hepatobiliary System & Pancreas	20	66%
Other Pneumonia	19	67%
Extnsv Proc Unrelat To Principal Diagnosis	19	68%
Craniotomy Except for Trauma	18	69%
Lymphoma & Nonacute Leukemia	16	70%
Maj Respiratory Infections & Inflammations	15	71%
Resp Syst Diagn w/ Vent Support 96+ Hours	13	72%
Cardiac Arrest	13	72%
Neonate BWT<500G	13	73%
Chronic Obstructive Pulmonary Disease	12	74%
Peripheral & Other Vascular Disorders	12	74%
Oth & Unspecified Gastrointestinal Hemorrhage	12	75%

Now consider primary ICD-10 diagnosis codes for those who died in hospital.

What is the take-home message? We are looking at cost, diagnoses summarized by 3M APR DRG, and diagnoses summarized by ICD-10 Primary. What can you deduce?

We see that for those who ultimately die in hospital, 54 percent of the average annual inpatient revenue collected per person antecedent to date of death ($93,474.02) is collected in the last seven days of life. Clearly, the last days are the most expensive.

Table 50. Primary ICD dx of in-hospital deaths 2017

ICD dx Primary	Count	Cum Pct
A41.9 Sepsis, unspecified organism	488	25%
I13.0-Hypertensive heart and chronic kidney disease with heart failure and stage 1 through st	52	27%
A41.89 Other specified sepsis	44	29%
A1.51-Sepsis due to Escherichia coli (e. coli)	34	31%
N17.9-Acute Kidney failure, unspecified	31	33%
A41.02-Sepsis due to methicillin resistant Staphylococcus Aureus	29	34%
I11.0-Hypertensive heart disease with heart failure	28	36%
A41.01-Sepsis due to methicillin susceptible Staphylococcus aureus	26	37%
I13.2-Hypertensive heart and chronic kidney disease with heart failure and with stage 5 chronic kidney	23	38%
J96.01-Acute respiratory failure with hypoxia	22	39%
J18.9-Pneumonia, unspecified organism	22	40%
I21.4-Non-ST elevation (NSTEMI) myocardial infarction	22	41%
A41.59-Other gram-negative sepsis	22	42%
K92.2-Gastrointestinal hemorrhage, unspecified	20	43%
A41.81- Sepsis due to Enterococcus	17	44%
Z38.00-Single liveborn infant, delivered vaginally	17	45%
C78.6-Secondary malignant neoplasm of retroperitoneum and peritoneum	16	46%
A41.52-Sepsis due to Pseudomonas	16	47%

C78.6 - Secondary malignant neoplasm of retroperitoneum and peritoneum	16	47%
I46.9 - Cardiac arrest, cause unspecified	15	48%
I21.3 - ST elevation (STEMI) myocardial infarction of unspecified site	14	49%
K70.31 - Alcoholic cirrhosis of liver with ascites	13	49%
K72.90 - Hepatic failure, unspecified without coma	12	50%
Z38.01 - Single liveborn infant, delivered by cesarean	12	51%
I61.8 - Other nontraumatic intracerebral hemorrhage	12	51%
I63.412 - Cerebral infarction due to embolism of left middle cerebral artery	11	52%
A41.4 - Sepsis due to anaerobes	11	52%
I63.512 - Cerebral infarction due to unspecified occlusion or stenosis of left middle cerebral artery	10	53%
C25.9 - Malignant neoplasm of pancreas, unspecified	10	53%
J44.0 - Chronic obstructive pulmonary disease with (acute) lower respiratory infection	10	54%
T81.4XXA - Infection following a procedure, initial encounter	10	54%
I21.09 - ST elevation (STEMI) myocardial infarction involving other coronary artery of anterior wall	9	55%
C22.0 - Liver cell carcinoma	9	55%
I21.19 - ST elevation (STEMI) myocardial infarction involving other coronary artery of inferior wall	9	56%
I47.2 - Ventricular tachycardia	9	56%
I63.9 - Cerebral infarction, unspecified	9	57%
I60.9 - Nontraumatic subarachnoid hemorrhage, unspecified	8	57%
I63.411 - Cerebral infarction due to embolism of right middle cerebral artery	8	57%
C79.31 - Secondary malignant neoplasm of brain	8	58%
B20 - Human immunodeficiency virus (HIV) disease	8	58%
I26.99 - Other pulmonary embolism without acute cor pulmonale	7	59%
J96.00 - Acute respiratory failure, unspecified whether with hypoxia or hypercapnia	7	59%
I61.9 - Nontraumatic intracerebral hemorrhage, unspecified	7	59%
G89.3 - Neoplasm related pain (acute) (chronic)	7	60%
J96.02 - Acute respiratory failure with hypercapnia	7	60%
N39.0 - Urinary tract infection, site not specified	7	60%
I50.23 - Acute on chronic systolic (congestive) heart failure	7	61%
C34.11 - Malignant neoplasm of upper lobe, right bronchus or lung	7	61%
R62.7 - Adult failure to thrive	7	61%
J44.1 - Chronic obstructive pulmonary disease with (acute) exacerbation	7	62%
C90.00 - Multiple myeloma not having achieved remission	7	62%
C78.00 - Secondary malignant neoplasm of unspecified lung	6	62%
C79.51 - Secondary malignant neoplasm of bone	6	63%
I26.09 - Other pulmonary embolism with acute cor pulmonale	6	63%
E11.51 - Type 2 diabetes mellitus with diabetic peripheral angiopathy without gangrene	6	63%
A41.50 - Gram-negative sepsis, unspecified	6	64%
K70.40 - Alcoholic hepatic failure without coma	6	64%
A40.3 - Sepsis due to Streptococcus pneumoniae	6	64%
E11.52 - Type 2 diabetes mellitus with diabetic peripheral angiopathy with gangrene	6	65%
K74.60 - Unspecified cirrhosis of liver	6	65%
J95.851 - Ventilator associated pneumonia	6	65%
I71.01 - Dissection of thoracic aorta	6	65%

Both the APR DRG and the ICD-10 review suggest that 25 percent of the diagnoses in the terminal hospitalization are sepsis related. A good deal of effort is underway in our institution and locally in our city to improve surveillance for rapid and aggressive intervention of septic shock. The hope, of course, is that by removing this proximal cause of death, we might be able to reduce mortality and cost. While it is reasonable, it is clearly possible that the septic shock is an indicator of the poor biologic substrate of the patient susceptible to sepsis and that the removal of this cause will just reveal another. This is yet to be determined.

How Would You Plan for the Use of a New Pharmaceutical Agent in Your LHS?

M anagement of end-stage renal disease is extremely costly with costs increasing exponentially as the disease progresses.[52] Moving from stage 4 to 5 (from a glomerular filtration rate range of 15–30 to 0–15 ml/min, respectively) is accompanied by the significant costs of developing a shunt for dialysis and instituting dialysis. In addition to dollar costs, there are significant costs in quality of life. The ability to delay progression particularly across this cutpoint of glomerular filtration rate is therefore important.

In 2019, a study of the drug Atrasentin[53] claimed to delay the progression of renal disease in type 2 diabetics aged 18–85, with an albumin:creatinine ratio in the 300–5,000 range.

As a learning health system, maintaining surveillance on options for health care optimization, we immediately undertook an assessment of our population to determine how many might be benefitted by the new medication once it would become available.

We provide the analytic steps using our population cohort builder, Clinical Looking Glass, to model the identification of the eligible patients in our population and then establish their natural history of renal function decay under our care. We thereby identify the basic capabilities required of any software system wishing to support core LHS objectives.

We first identify the number of unique patients in our primary care MMG group who had an outpatient visit in 2016 and were aged 18–85 (N=140,726).

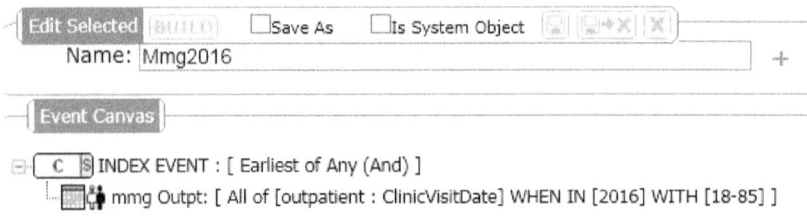

Figure 48. Cohort of MMG primary care patients ages 18–85, 2016 (N=140,726)

Now require that these have evidence of diabetes with a HbA1c ≥ 6.5 in the antecedent 1,825 days (5 years), N=34,736.

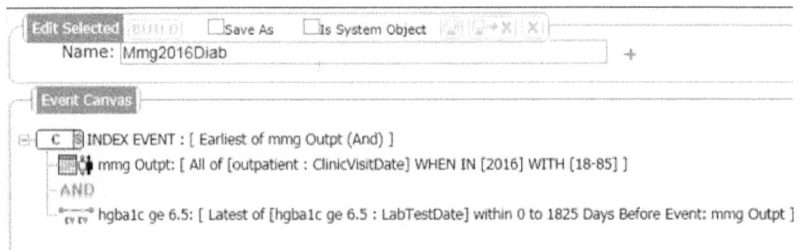

Figure 49. MMG primary care diabetic patients age 18–85, 2016 (N=34,736)

1. Now eliminate those with reported type 1 diabetes by ICD-10 in 2016 to leave us with patients with Diabetes Type 2 (N=34,002).

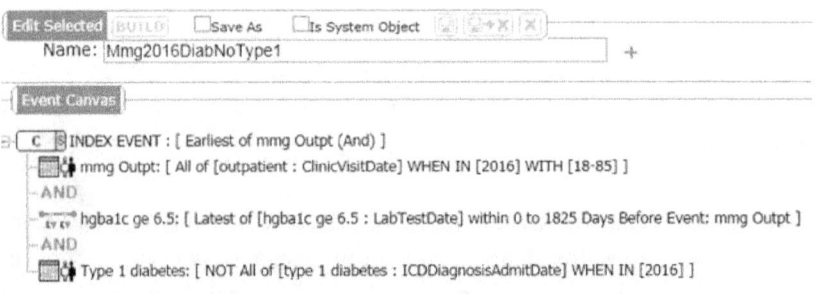

Figure 50. MMG primary care type 2 diabetic patients age 18–85, 2016 (N=34,002)

2. Now require an Estimated Glomerular Filtration Rate (EGFR) first using the equation for non-African Americans (calculated for everyone) [15–30 ml/

min), N=20,369. Recapitulating the analysis using the equation for estimated GFR for African American calculation finds N=20,395. For the purpose of the calculations going forward, we will use the equation for all persons who are not African Americans.

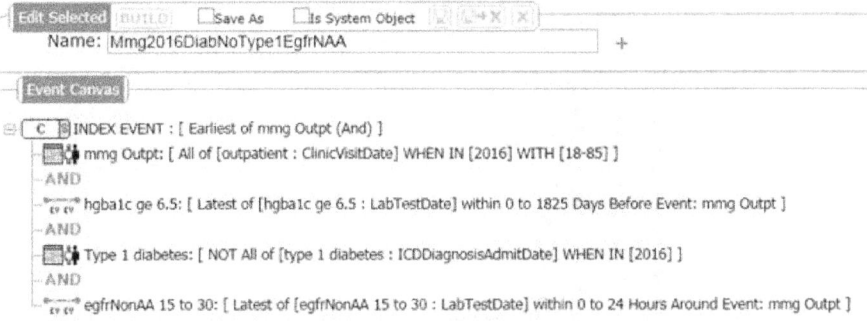

Figure 51. MMG primary care type 2 diabetic patients age 18–85 estimated GFR 15–30, 2016 (N=20,369)

Now use the non-AA group and require a Urine Albumin to Creatinine Ratio (UACR) of 300–5000 mg/g (N=822).

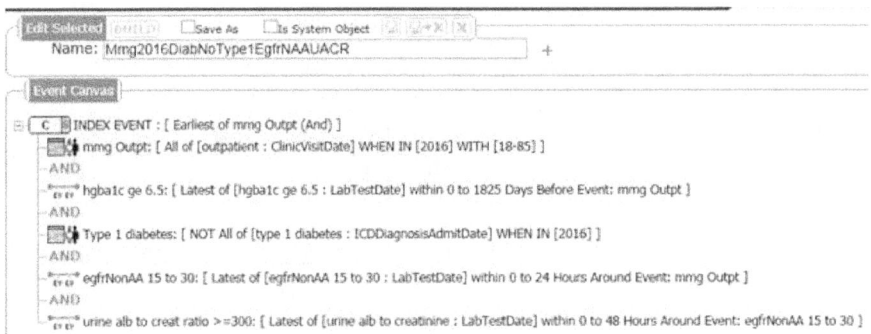

Figure 52. MMG primary care type 2 diabetic patients age 18–85
estimated GFR 15–30 alb/cr≥300, 2016 (N=822)

Having built a cohort of stage 4 type 2 diabetics with proteinuria, we now will perform a time-to-outcome analysis where the outcome is achieving an estimated GFR of 0–15 ml/min. The crossing of this critical threshold has significant cost and morbidity implications.

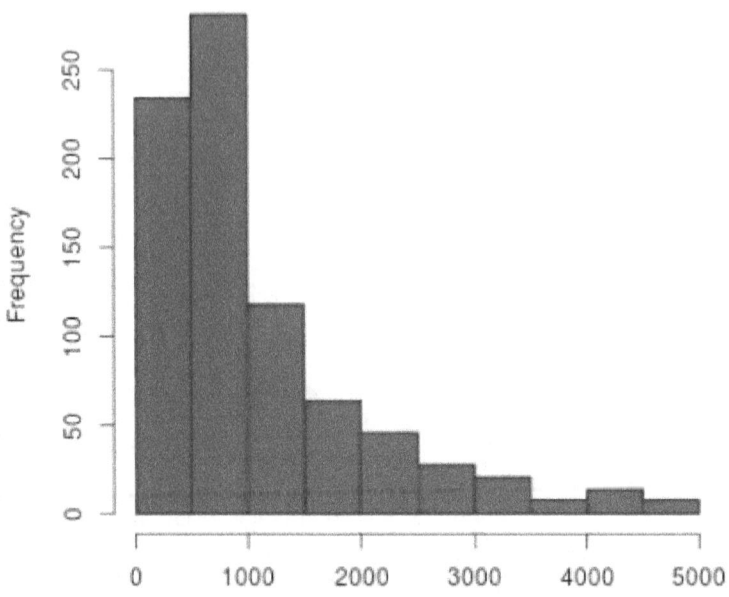

Figure 53. Histogram for urine albumin/creatinine ratio

Mean	Median	Variance	Standard deviation	Valid N
1,124	774	892,838	945	822
Minimum	1st Quartile	Median	3rd Quartile	Maximum
300	473	774	1,406	4,997

Figure 54. Summary urine albumin/creatinine ratio

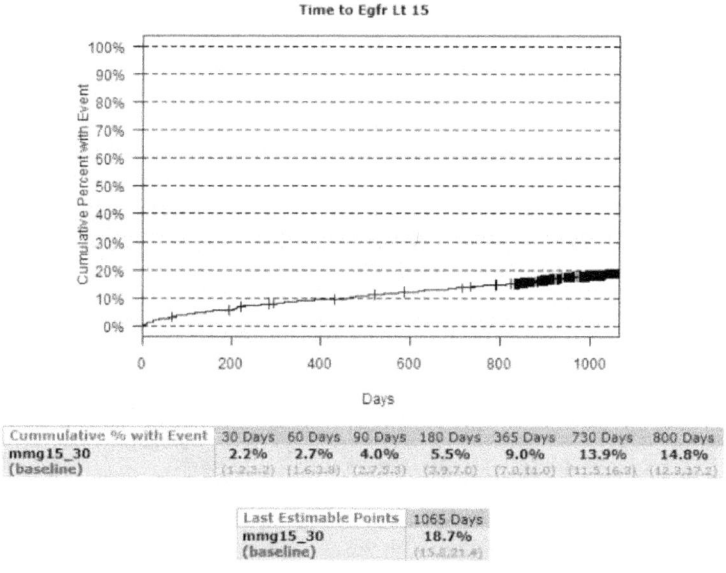

Figure 55. Time to outcome of GFR<15 ml/min criteria (Clinical Looking Glass)

Sex	Male #(%)	Female #(%)	Unknown #(%)
mmg15_30 (baseline)	422 (51.34)	400 (48.66)	0 (0)

Age Percentiles					(median)				
	Minimum	5th	10th	25th	50th	75th	90th	95th	100th
mmg15_30 (baseline)	23	44	47	55	63	71	78	80	84

Figure 56. Sex and age tables

All told, 146 patients crossed the threshold. You WILL notice that at 30 days, we have 2.2% crossing the threshold, suggesting that the original eGFR estimate was not stable.

Over the ensuing days to day 365, 9% crossed the threshold. Horizontal marks are placed at censorship, which, prior to 800 days, is due to death. With this real-world local information, we can plan for the impact of new medications claiming specific rates of progression reduction and build models of costs and savings to develop and maintain intervention programs.

Real Hospital Epidemiology Surveillance: Critical Capability of a Learning Health System

Ongoing Nosocomial Roommate Transmission of C. difficile Detected by Advanced Cohort Analytics

Background

For more than three decades, outbreaks of infectious diarrhea have been recognized in hospitalized patients.[54-57] Care for US patients with *Clostridial difficile* infection (CDI) is estimated to cost between 436 million and 3.2 billion dollars per year.[58] Reports of the successful use of gloves to interrupt nosocomial transmission[59] and demonstrations of the degree of effectiveness of different hand hygiene strategies for the elimination of *C. difficile* spores[60] contribute to the suspicion that much of the increasing prevalence of CDI[61] is a consequence of chronic low-level, intra-institutional spread with occasional exacerbations manifested as outbreaks.

A number of papers using advanced genetic technologies have failed to show a large component of intra-institutional spread.[62,63] Walker and colleagues used molecular typing and epidemiologic linkage to hospital wards (20–30 beds in 4–6 bedded bays) but not rooms, and they failed to find at the ward level a relationship between location and linked cases.[64] This is despite the fact that Hamel[65] demonstrated that an increased number of roommates was a risk factor for *C. difficile* transmission, and Duberke[66] found that ward-level high *C. difficile* prevalence was a risk factor in a case control study.

The creation of cohorts using EMRs now permits us to build in-room *C. difficile*-exposed cohorts and controls and then use advanced statistical methods to establish the presence of ongoing intra-institutional transmission of *C. difficile*. In this report, we will demonstrate the technique that we suspect could ultimately be used to monitor the quality of infection control efforts.

Method
Population
Montefiore Medical Center (MMC) includes three adult hospitals and one children's hospital with 1,491 beds in the Bronx, NY. In 2013, 492,993 people received inpatient or outpatient care at least once in this system, which resides in a borough with 1.4 million people. In 2013, MMC saw 89,900 admissions. All patients admitted to one of the hospitals of the Montefiore Medical System between January 1, 2011 and January 1, 2014 were eligible for study inclusion.

An EMR system supported both inpatient and outpatient medical care. Its data were consolidated incrementally on a daily basis in a data warehouse with an analytic engine, Clinical Looking Glass, and were available to build and analyze deidentified cohorts.

C. difficile Case Definition
Patient stools evaluated for *C. difficile* in the course of standard clinical care underwent the following protocol. Stools were tested by ELISA for glutamate dehydrogenase (Wampole® C.diff Chek 60 [Techlab, Blacksburg, VA]). If they came back as antigen positive, confirmatory tests included Wampole ToxA/B II from 2009 to 2011 (>0.8ng Toxin A, >2.5 ng Toxin B) and Wampole ToxA/B QuikChek 2012 to present (>0.63ng Toxin A, >1.25ng Toxin B). If the toxin was not found, the toxin B gene was sought using Cepheid Xpert C. difficile/Epi (Cepeheid, Sunnyvale, CA) for the detection of toxin B gene sequences and for the presumptive ID of the 027/NAP1/B1 strain of toxigenic *C. difficile*. For the purpose of this study, a patient was considered a case of *C. difficile* when either the toxin or the gene sequence was found to be positive.

Cohort Definition

Potential Infectious Source

From 1/1/2011 to 1/1/2014, we built a cohort of hospitalized patients who were C. difficile positive for the first time in the MMC laboratory. These patients were considered potential sources of infection for their roommates.

Exposed Cohort Defined

We identified all patients who were in the same room as a member of the potential source cohort within 24–72 hours of the laboratory test diagnosing the source patient. This 24–72-hour window was defined as the period of infectivity. To be included in the exposed cohort, a patient had to occupy the same room as the infected source during the period of infectivity for at least 24 hours and no more than 72 hours.

Control Cohorts Defined

We identified two control groups labeled "before" and "after." The before-control cohort patients spent 24–72 hours in the same room as the source patient but did so 60–100 days before the source patient entered the room. The after-control cohort spent 24–72 hours 60–100 days after the source patient left the room. The control groups, therefore, shared similarities that inhered to the location of the bed, service, and clinical and support staff.

We eliminated from both control groups those patients who had already been included in the exposed cohort. We then removed from the after-control group those patients who had been included in the before-control group. The resulting three groups contained unique members.

During the analysis stage, we eliminated from all three groups those with evidence of MMC laboratory-detected CDI in the preceding 90 days.

Outcome Measure Statistical Analysis

The outcome was laboratory-detected C. difficile. The conversion of an exposed or control group member into a case was summarized as crude cumulative incidence using the complement of the Kaplan-Meier statistic.

Multivariate analytic methods of risk and logistic regression[67,68] evaluated the effect of *C. difficile* roommate exposure on the development *of C. difficile* in the ensuing 90 days.

Variables considered included those known to be associated with the development of *C. difficile*: the use of a proton pump inhibitor (PPI), the use of antibiotics during hospitalization, the use of antibiotics in the outpatient prior to index hospitalization, age, and illness severity as measured by a modification of the Charlson Comorbidity Index[43,44,46] based upon all inpatient, outpatient, and emergency department diagnoses available from care delivered at Montefiore in the preceding year. APR-DRG weight (3M Salt Lake City, Utah), a metric of resource utilization in the index hospitalization, was also considered as an adjuster, as were the impact of H2 blockers, gender, race (not white), and ethnicity (Hispanic). The Hosmer-Lemeshow goodness of fit statistic[69-71] was used to test for logistic model adequacy.

To obtain an estimate of the absolute risk of exposure in the exposed accounting for the variables used in the risk regression model, the following procedure was followed. All exposed patients were identified, and their individual risk was predicted by the risk regression model first calculated with the exposure variable set to "exposed" and then calculated with the exposure variable set to "not exposed." The average calculated risk difference was obtained by subtracting the two calculated risks for each patient and averaging those differences. This average was therefore the calculated risk difference due to exposure. A 95% confidence interval was calculated using the approach of a large-sample normal distribution of errors from two populations. We calculated the number needed to harm as a meaningful way of expressing the risk of roommate exposure. The number needed to harm is the reciprocal of the average risk difference[72,73] and provides the number of patients needed to be exposed to a CDI patient to generate one new case of CDI.

Statistical modeling procedures were implemented and integrated in R by Scry Health (New Haven, CT) in a package we developed for our own institutional use and soon to be available as a commercial package.

Hospital-Acquired C. difficile

Hospital-acquired *C. difficile* infection (HACDI) was defined as modified by Curry[74] who had modified McDonald.[75] Patients were eliminated from consideration as hospital acquired if they had an MMC laboratory-documented CDI in the preceding six months.

Once the exclusion criterion was met, the inclusion criteria was dependent upon whether the positive *C. difficile* test occurred within the first two days of the current hospitalization. For patients diagnosed in the first two days of the current hospitalization, the attribution of the *C. difficile* to MMC required an admission to Montefiore in the preceding 12 weeks without EMR evidence of another health care institution exposure (hospital, nursing home, or rehabilitation facility). Health care institution exposure was established by EMR evidence of admission from such an institution on the present admission or admission from or discharge to such an institution on a previous MMC admission.

Patients diagnosed from day three onward without MMC laboratory evidence of *C. difficile* in the preceding six months were considered hospital acquired even if they did not have previous MMC inpatient exposure.

Our definition differs from Curry's in that we did not require the documentation of clinical signs and symptoms of *C. difficile* to establish a case, and no patient interview was undertaken to search for health care institution exposure.

Results

From January 1, 2011 through January 1, 2014, MMC had 267,639 admissions. There were 3,912 admissions of patients with laboratory evidence of CDI. Of these, 2,344 patients were diagnosed for the first time in the MMC laboratory. 3,900 patients were exposed to potential source patients within 24–72 hours of their laboratory diagnosis and spent 24–72 hours in the same room as the potential source. 10,600 controls were identified 60–100 days prior to the potential source case, and 8,218 controls were identified 60–100 days after the source case. The 90-day crude cumulative incidence of *C. difficile* for exposed, before-control, and after-control patients was 5.3% (4.5,6.0), 2.1% (1.8,2.4), and 1.8% (1.5,2.1), respectively $P<.00001$ (Table 51).

Table 51. Crude cumulative incidence C. difficile

	By 15 days	By 30 days	By 60 days	By 90 days
C. difficile-exposed*	2.6% (2.1,3.1)	3.3% (2.7,3.8)	4.5% (3.8,5.2)	5.3% (4.5,6.0)

Before control**	1.4% (1.2,1.6)	1.6% (1.3,1.8)	1.9% (1.7,2.2)	2.1% (1.8,2.4)
After control***	1.2% (1.0,1.4)	1.4% (1.1,1.6)	1.7% (1.4,2.0)	1.8% (1.5,2.1)

*C. difficile-exposed: patients exposed as roommates for 24–72 hours to potential source CDI patients.
** Before control: patients admitted to the same room as potential source patients 60 days before the potential source patients.
*** After control: patients admitted to the same room as potential source patients 60 days after the potential source patients.

We collapsed both the before and after controls into a single control group and found that exposure to a roommate with C. difficile significantly increased the unadjusted odds of developing CDI (Odds Ratio 2.38, 95% CI 1.95–2.90, p<.001).

Categorical and continuous variable summaries revealed that the C. difficile-exposed group was older and sicker (by Charlson and APR-DRG) than their control counterparts (Table 52, Table 53) with an adjusted Odds Ratio of 1.41, 95% CI 1.15–1.74, p=.001.

Table 52. Categorical variables

	Potential Infectious Source	C. difficile-Exposed	Control*
Number**	2,149	3,649	18,589
Male (%)	889 (41%)	1,604 (44%)	7,944 (42%)
Race not white (%)	1,642 (76%)	2,896 (79%)	15,091 (81%)
Ethnicity Hispanic (%)	812 (38%)	1,411 (39%)	7,779 (42%)
Proton pump inhibitor	1,185 (55%)	1,944 (53%)	6,732 (36%)
H2 blocker	469 (22%)	1,141 (31%)	3,363 (18%)
Antibiotic during hospitalization	1,706 (79%)	2,377 (65%)	8,891(48%)
Antibiotic within 30 days before hospitalization	296 (14%)	247 (7%)	1,324 (7%)

*Control: patients admitted to the same room as potential source patients 60 days before or after the potential source patients.
**Number of patients who could report on all the variables (Table 52, Table 53).

Table 53. Continuous variables

	Potential Infectious Source	C. difficile Exposed	Control*
Age			
10th Percentile	37	35	24
25th Percentile	55	50	44
50th Percentile	68	63	59
75th Percentile	80	76	73
90th Percentile	88	84	83
Charlson Score			
10th Percentile	1	0	0
25th Percentile	3	2	1
50th Percentile	6	4	3
75th Percentile	9	7	6
90th Percentile	11	10	9
APR-DRG weight**			
10th Percentile	0.91	0.63	0.46
25th Percentile	1.39	0.95	0.58
50th Percentile	2.67	1.89	0.87
75th Percentile	3.46	3.39	1.58
90th Percentile	7.14	6.29	3.25
Length of Stay			
10th Percentile	4	2	1
25th Percentile	7	4	2
50th Percentile	12	7	3
75th Percentile	19	14	5
90th Percentile	30	23	11
Number of Previous Discharges			
10th Percentile	0	0	0
25th Percentile	0	0	0
50th Percentile	1	0	0
75th Percentile	2	2	1
90th Percentile	4	3	3

*Control Group includes both the *before* and *after* *Control* group

**APR-DRG: risk-adjustment methodology of 3M corporation collapsing ICD-9 diagnoses during the inpatient stay into coherent severity-adjusted single-summary diagnosis group representing the hospitalization with a notion of resource consumption weight used as a clinical severity proxy in the analysis.

Repeating the analysis with a risk regression yielded a C. *difficile* roommate exposure relative risk of 1.36, 95% CI 1.19–1.55, p<.01) (Table 54).

Table 54 Relative risk of developing C. difficile

Variable	Relative Risk (95% confidence Interval)*
Exposed Yes vs. No	1.36 (1.19,1.55)
PPI	1.37 (1.20,1.58)
Antibiotic prescribed in hospital	3.15 (2.47,4.02)
Age	1.008 (1.004,1.012)
Length of stay	1.006 (1.004,1.008)
Charlson	1.05 (1.03,1.07)
Discharges in preceding year	1.10 (1.08,1.12)

*all p≤.0001

As shown in previous studies, the use of a proton pump inhibitor and in-hospital antibiotics were associated with increased odds for the development of C. *difficile*. Length of stay, increasing age, and number of discharges in the preceding year were also significant risk factors. H2 blockers use, gender, race, ethnicity, and outpatient antibiotic prescription in the preceding 30 days to admission and APR-DRG weight for the index admission were not significant risk factors (C statistic 0.762). The Hosmer Lemeshow goodness-of-fit statistic p=.11 did not reject the logistic model.

Using the risk regression model for the exposed patients, we calculated an average risk difference due to roommate C. *difficile* exposure among the exposed of .01, 95% CI .002–.019, p=.014. The number needed to harm for the exposed was 97 (95% CI 54–486). Ninety-seven patients had to be exposed to a roommate with C. *difficile* to generate a single new case of C. *difficile*.

Hospital-acquired C. *difficile* rates provided as number diagnosed per 10,000 patient days were 13.5, 12.6, and 13.1 for the years 2011, 2012, and 2013, respectively. These rates dropped to 7.0, 7.1, and 7.3, respectively, when we ignored any case detected after the second day of hospitalization for patients who spent any time in another health care institution in the preceding 84 days.

Discussion

Sharing a room with a patient with *C. difficile* in our hospital increased a patient's risk of CDI by 36% even after adjusting for other variables known to be associated with infection.

Compared to the *C. difficile*-exposed roommates, the control group was considerably younger and less sick by the criteria of the Charlson Comorbidity Index, length of stay, and APR-DRG weight. We were surprised by this finding as we anticipated that controls drawn from the same rooms and floors as the *C. difficile* exposed should have had characteristics indistinguishable from the controls.

One possible explanation could have been conscious cohorting of patients by staff keeping sicker patients together for the convenience of managing them. Even if this were a plausible explanation in principle, it would have been impractical. MMC bed occupancy was high, and bed availability for ER assignment was a near-random event, except in priority cases of infection control. As soon as a bed became available for occupancy, it was filled by the next patient waiting in the emergency room. Routine cohorting would have required a luxury of bed capacity or time that did not exist. If the initial bed assignment from the emergency department did not result in sick patient cohorting, could there have been a post admission process routinely reorganizing bed assignments within the floor population? This too seemed to be unreasonable to those who actually work on the hospital floors.

We think that part of the explanation may be found in this set of logical syllogisms.

Greater length of stay ➜ implies greater chance of exposure to a source patient

Greater length of stay ➜ implies a patient who is older and sicker

Therefore, The *C. difficile*-exposed group is composed of older and sicker patients than controls drawn from the same room at a different time.

No special conscious cohorting was required to achieve the observed functional enrichment of sicker patients in the *C. difficile*-exposed group.

Another factor biasing the *C. difficile* exposed to sicker patients than the controls was the way patients were assigned to mutually exclusive groups. A patient in the exposed group was removed from both control groups. If removed from the before-control group, the exposed group would have been given a patient with one more discharge than it would have had had it been included in the before-control group. If removed from the after-control group, the exposed group would have gotten a patient with one fewer admission than would have been given to the after-control group, but the patient it had received was predestined to be sick enough for yet another admission so he was of the sicker variety. If a patient was in both control groups, his representative admission would have been that of the before-control group and therefore with at least one fewer discharge.

If we believe that patients with more antecedent discharges are sicker, this process selected the less severe admission of the two possible in both controls. Because we are concerned that the indicia of sickliness might predispose patients to manifest *C. difficile* clinically, we built multivariate analyses to adjust for these differences and continued to see a significant impact of exposure on the development of *C. difficile*.

We were conservative in our choice of potential source patients. We allowed only the first-time diagnosed *C. difficile* patients (2,344 [60%]) to be considered as source patients of the total prevalent CDI admissions of 3,912. We did this in the hope that incident patients would be more homogeneous in terms of shedding without suppression by antibiotics. If, in fact, the ignored 40% were shedding and exposing patients, then some of those we identified as unexposed were misclassified, improperly shrinking the calculated relative risk and risk difference. The misclassification biased against the direction of our observations, making our observed significant relative risk of exposure 1.36 and absolute risk difference of 1% underestimate their true values. The number of exposed patients needed to generate a single new CDI case would have been even smaller than the observed 97.

To contextualize our environment, we compared the MMC rates of hospital-acquired *C. difficile* infection (HACDI) to those reported by the University of Pittsburgh Medical Center. Between 2006 and 2012, UPMC reported HACDI rates of 5.6 per 10,000 patient days.[74] MMC rates were 12.6–13.5 per 10,000 patient days in 2011–2013. If we had ignored any HACDI case with evidence of admission to some non MMC health care entity in the preceding 84 days, then the MMC rates would have been reduced to an average of 7.1 per 10,000 patient days. Keep in mind that our rates did not benefit by the taking of a clinical history, which would have disqualified patients without multiple loose stools or with a history of previous health care site exposure unrecorded in the MMC EMR—inclusion criteria of the Pittsburgh study.

As a quality marker for infection control practice, *C. difficile* is far from an ideal indicator. Since we know of asymptomatic carriage,[54] it might be inferred that *C. difficile* could have a long incubation period waiting for antibiotic suppression of normal gut flora or host debilitation to flower into disease. The possibility of transmission from affiliated nursing homes and rehabilitation facilities further complicates certain attribution.

Nosocomial transmission of C. *difficile* is underestimated by our study's case definition, which relies upon clinician suspicion of disease to order case-finding laboratory tests. A prospective culture study of 59% of the admitted patients to a medical ward (N=428) revealed that 52 of the 83 (63%) incident culture-positive patients were asymptomatic.[54]

Since the transmission of C. *difficile* to a relatively healthy roommate without antibiotic or proton pump inhibitor therapy could be clinically silent, we suspect that a routine study of all roommates would have demonstrated rates of transmission far in excess of what we reported.

Conclusion

Exposure to a roommate with newly diagnosed C. *difficile* is a risk factor for developing C. *difficile* infection. Automated surveillance of exposed and control cohorts created from data in the EMR with advanced statistical modeling can provide a deeper understanding of the local dynamics of in-hospital disease transmission with the potential to evaluate the effectiveness of local interventions.

What Additional Software Tools Are Required to Support Hospital Epidemiology?

Assuming you have read the preceding chapter and understood the power of infectious disease exposure surveillance in a hospital, consider the capability you would have to build in your cohort builder to accomplish this task. Who in the institution with resources could bring a team together to do this, and why would they? In this chapter, I will describe at a conceptual level what the module that accomplished this task had to consider. You should ask yourself the following questions:

1. What sort of capabilities would need to be intrinsic to your initial cohort builder tool to allow the addition of this capability?
2. Who would be incentivized to build, maintain, and train the use of this tool?
3. What would the source of funding be?
4. Can you imagine a federal grant that would fund one institution to build a tool that had to be tailored to the specific information system of the grantee? The grantee would first establish the appropriate data flows to feed the analytic and then maintain that flow through the frequent data corruptions and disruptions promulgated by the EMR vendors to serve their internal upgrade needs in blissful disregard for downstream reporting and analytic consequences outside of their product.

Consider the reigning model of analytics in hospitals.[3]

- Use some sort of filter on a limited subset of hospital data to find patients with a few attributes. These cohorts are lists of names but not true analytic objects that support subsequent temporal analyses.[3]
- Dashboards report on fixed predetermined questions to support reimbursement for quality.
- A few scattered PhDs and SQL programmers pull data from a data repository to perform a "one-off" study that is not easily operationally reproduced. This model supported by federal academic grants leaves nothing operationally useful behind.

Background

Investigation of infectious disease exposure in a hospital often requires identifying those patients who shared a common room with an infectious patient. The user must know the date the patient became infectious.

Practically speaking, the infection control coordinator would create a cohort of infected patients in a spreadsheet recording for each patient an index date (when his infection could be communicable) and the end date (the date he no longer is considered infectious for the purpose of this analysis).

The identification of patients exposed to members of the cohort is important for the purpose of prophylaxis, observation, or isolation. While it is not possible to build a generic ventilation-based exposure analytic, since this requires a detailed understanding of air ventilation in the hospital, we are able to build an analytic that provides the user with a list of those patients who shared time in the same room with the index patient.

This analytic provides the user with a list of patients who shared the same space and gives the capability of building a cohort of these patients for use in other modules of Clinical Looking Glass. The analytic also provides the user with the ability to build control cohorts, people exposed to the same hospital room at a time when the infectious patient was not yet there. The control cohort can have dwell time in the same room either before or after the source patient. The control cohort can be used to evaluate the relationship between exposure and downstream outcomes.

Concept of Exposure to an Infected Patient

To conceptualize exposure, see Figure 57 below and read the discussion that follows.

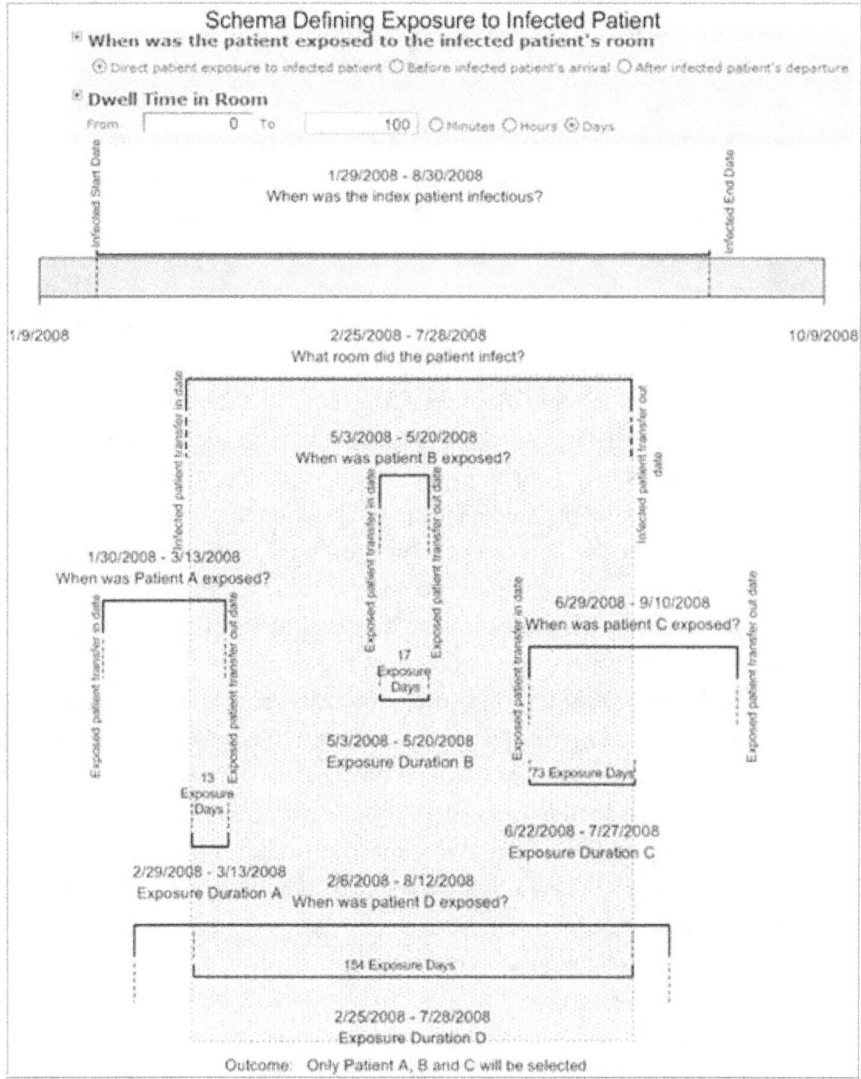

Figure 57. Mechanism for identifying patients exposed to infected patient

You must do the following:

1. Identify the infectious patients. The user must tell the computer for each infectious patient the date of communicability as well as when he was no longer infectious. This is accomplished by identifying a cohort of patients and using the index date of each patient member as the date of communicability onset. In typical CLG fashion, we will define the duration of follow-up communicability by risk window, use end date, and/or calendar date from/to, yielding the combined and therefore most restricted duration as the duration of communicability. The spreadsheets produced from the analytic will identify the start date of infectivity in the source patient as Infected Start Date. Similarly, the end date of infectivity will be Infected End Date.

2. Define the time window that the infected patient spent in a room in the communicable state. This dwell time constitutes the time during which the infection could be spread to other members of the room. The start time for the room being considered infectious as a result of the source patient is called Infected Patient Transfer-in Date. Similarly, the date of departure of the source infected patient from the room or spontaneous termination of his infectivity is called the Infected Patient Transfer-out Date. These dates are automatically determined by the smart report engine, which looks to see what rooms the source infected patient occupied during the period of communicability of his disease.

3. Identify which patients were exposed to the communicable source patient. These patients spent time in a bed in the same room as the infected (communicable) source patient when the communicable patient was there. You might want to require a certain duration of overlap time before the exposed patient is to be considered exposed (dwell time). Clinical Looking Glass will allow you to specify a duration of time from/to hours spent in overlap. An overlap of 0 minutes is an instantaneous communicability upon entering the communicable patient's room.

4. Develop control groups by requiring a specific dwell time in the infected patient's room either
    a. before his arrival into the room in an infected communicable state or
    b. after the infected patient departed the room or was declared noninfectious (transfer-out date).

Method

Left-click on Smart Report, then left-click on the plus sign in front of ad hoc, and then left-click on Infectious Disease Exposure smart report and expand the screen by clicking the Expand All button.

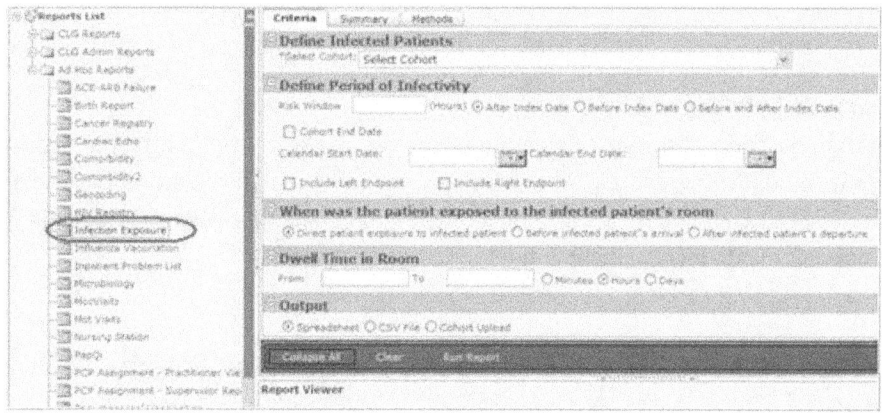

Figure 58. Link to Infection Exposure report

Define Infectious Patients

Define the period during which time exposure to the patient will result in the transmission of the disease. The period of infectivity always starts from the index date of the infected patient.

Risk Window (Hours)

Identify the duration in hours from the index date that your infectious patient is able to infect people in his hospital room. You can choose the direction of the hours as After, Before, or Before and After the Index Date.

Cohort End Date

Use the cohort end date associated with the cohort to terminate the period of infectivity.

Calendar Start/Stop Date

Use the Calendar Start/Stop date to restrict the period of infectivity.

The most restricted period of infectivity is the result of applying the rules the user has chosen in the risk window, cohort end date, and calendar start/stop date.

Include Left/Right Endpoint

If the user chooses not to include the endpoints, the query will subtract a second from the date:time and include up to and including that time-second date:time. Exclude Left Endpoint means including Left Endpoint date:time +1 sec. Exclude Right Endpoint means include Right Endpoint date:time -1 second.

When Was the Patient Exposed to the Infected Patient's Room?

Direct Patient Exposure to Infected Patient

This is the usual infection-control question and is the default. This option identifies the patients who were exposed to the infected patient's room when the infected patient was in the room. This means that the detected patients shared the room when the infected patient was there.

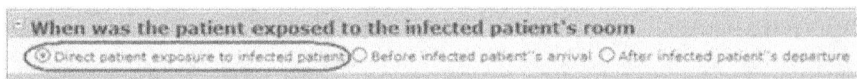

Figure 59. Direct exposure

For patients who are to be used as controls who were exposed to the room in question either before or after the infectious person left the room, we need to create an interval during which the exposure time is qualifying. This exposure time is an interval of days, hours, and minutes that either precede the arrival of the infected person or follow the departure of the infected person.

Before the Infected Patient's Arrival

This is the way to develop a control (nonexposed group of patients) who were exposed to the room before the infectious patient entered.

After the Infected Patient's Departure

This is the way to develop a control (nonexposed group of patients) who were exposed to the room after the infectious patient left the room or became noninfectious, whichever came first. If there is no end date, then you must use the date the infected patient departed from the room as the start point.

Dwell Time in Room

For patients with direct exposure to the infectious patient, this is the amount of time the patient must spend in the room with the infected patient to qualify as exposed. You provide the minimum exposure time to the maximum exposure time.

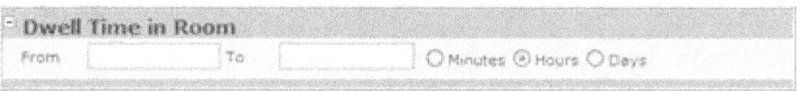

Figure 60. Dwell time in room

Similarly, for control groups, it is the amount of time spent in the room that the infected patient will either in the future be occupying or in the past occupied.

These are the outcomes if you had chosen the following.

During the Infected Patient's Stay

The dwell time in room will define the minimum to maximum exposure that will qualify a patient for being exposed. If you choose 0 to some large number, it will qualify overlap of a single second to as long as the largest number but no longer.

Before the Infected Patient's Arrival

The program will only qualify patients who spend the range of time inputted by the user in advance of the infected patient entering the room. Since there is no exposure to the infected patient directly, this is a form of a control group.

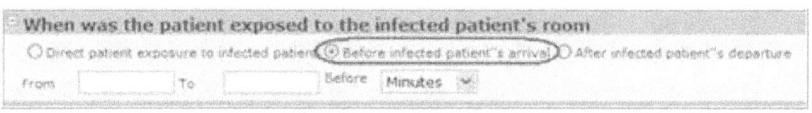

Figure 61. Exposed before infected patients' arrival

The user must inform Clinical Looking Glass the duration of time before the infected patient arrived in the room during which a control patient must dwell. The user must tell Clinical Looking Glass the minimum number of minutes/hours/days before to the maximum number of minutes/hours/days before the infected person's entry into the room when the unexposed patient could qualify as a control.

Since the exposure to the infected person's room was before the infected patient entered the room, the eligible time period when a control patient could be identified is calculated from the infected patient's arrival in the room (Infected Person's Transfer-in Date) backward in time to the minimum and maximum duration above.

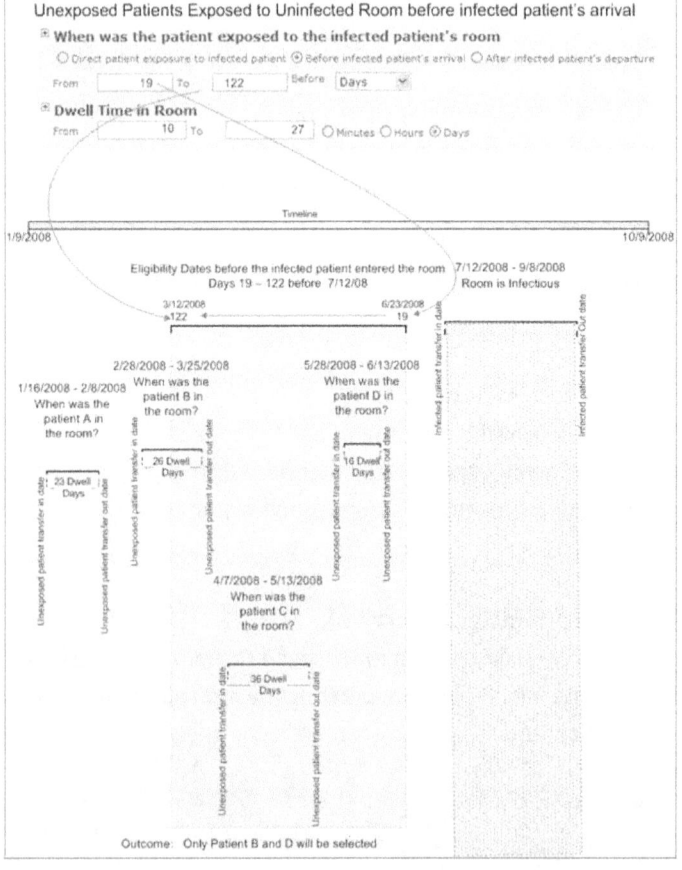

Figure 62. Selection mechanism for unexposed patients exposed to
uninfected room before infected patient's arrival

After the Infected Patient Departed

The program will only qualify patients who spend dwell time in the duration of time inputted by the user after the departure of the infected patient from the room. Since there is no exposure to the infected patient directly, this is a form of a control group.

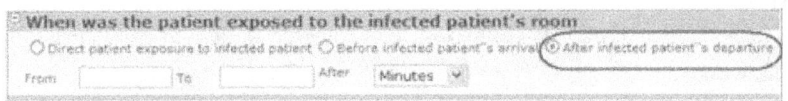

Figure 63. Exposed after infected patients' departure

Since the exposure to the infected person's room was after the infected patient left the room or lost infectivity, the designated duration during which the exposure time (dwell time) would be eligible would be calculated from the date:time of the departure of the infected patient from the room or of the spontaneous resolution of the patient's infectivity if he is still in the room but noninfectious (Infected Person's Transfer-out Date) until the minimum and maximum of the duration entered above.

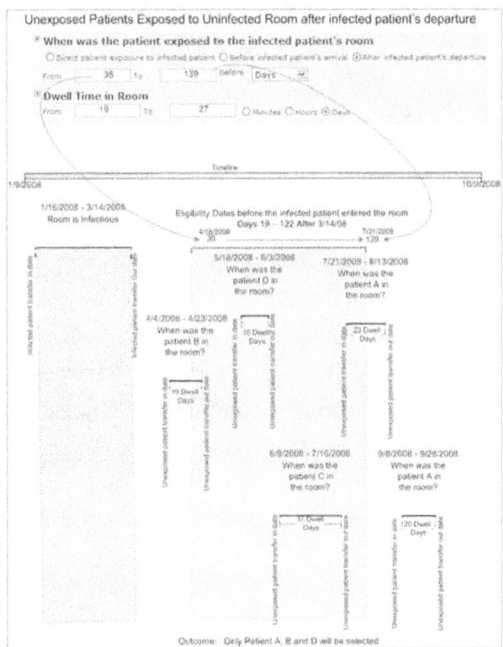

Figure 64. Selection mechanism for unexposed patients exposed to uninfected room after infected patient's departure

From/To (Minutes, Hours, Days)
This allows you to demand the amount of room dwell time.

Output
If you have chosen direct patient exposure to infected patient as exposure, consider the following:

1. The spreadsheet or CSV option will include every exposure to every member of the infected cohort each time there is an exposure. If the exposed patient is exposed twice in two different rooms, there will be two rows in the spreadsheet summarizing the two distinct exposures.
2. The cohort option will only include the first exposure setting the index date of the exposed as the date:time of first exposure.

The output will include patients who were located in the room of the index patient with either overlapping time in the room or no overlap time.

Required Capabilities
This analytic required a number of important capabilities.

1. The ability to either create cohorts in the application itself or importantly to upload a list with a medical record number, the date:time of communicability start (index date), and a third column with the end date for communicability.
2. The ability to move this defining cohort into the exposure study.
3. The ability to specify all the time conditions defining the nature of the exposure to the room and to infectious patients for the cases.

A Learning Health System Can Learn New Science from the EMR: Diabetes as Caused by Statins—The Choice of Sugar or Death

Abstract

Atorvastatin therapy has been associated with the development of diabetes but at the same time has been proven in specific populations to save lives in randomized controlled trials. Clinicians are challenged to contextualize the risks and benefits of this therapy.

Using 10 years of electronic medical data from a health care delivery system seeing more than 500,000 unique patients annually, we identify two cohorts of patients newly started on atorvastatin and simvastatin using the simvastatin group as a control to determine the relative risk of diabetes and death.

In the course of the paper, we explore the potential of big data to guide practice decisions using concepts not normally so explicitly employed in observational studies: intention to treat, bias in service of inference, and the use of a somewhat counterintuitive control to attenuate confounding by indication. Managing differential sensitivity to fact of death, due to the deterioration of the publicly available Social Security death tapes, through a matching strategy will also be discussed. This case study will demonstrate the potential of big data to answer a tough, practical, real-world clinical practice question and define the tools and effort that meaningful inference extraction will require.

Introduction

Atorvastatin therapy has been associated with the development of diabetes,[76-81] but at the same time, it is known to be lifesaving in randomized controlled trials[82,83] and in a recent observational case control study in type 2 diabetics.[84] Patients who have developed diabetes while prescribed atorvastatin are being besieged by lawyers asking them to participate in lawsuits against pharmaceutical manufacturers. In the current litigious climate, clinicians in practice must contextualize risks and make formal recommendations. In this paper, we demonstrate how a focused question and the appropriate use of analytics of big data available in EMRs can help clinicians draw inferences for decision making based upon real-world experience.

The trade-off that must be evaluated is between the development of diabetes and whatever benefit the drug has for preventing death. Presumably, if the drug causes diabetes but prevents death, most patients would choose the benefit of longer life. Being able to tell a patient of the experience of patients like them in their own community should be useful in a discussion of risks/benefits.

Methods
Population

Montefiore Medical Center is composed of 3 adult hospitals and one children's hospital with 1,492 beds in the Bronx, NY. In addition, primary care is provided in 21 outpatient clinics with 2.5 million annual outpatient visits (all types). In 2010, 500,000 unique individuals received inpatient or outpatient care at least once in this system, which resides in a borough with 1.3 million people.

All patients age 40 or older seen in the Montefiore Medical System between January 1, 2005 through January 1, 2014 were eligible for consideration in this study.

An EMR system supports both inpatient and outpatient medical care. The data are consolidated incrementally on a daily basis in a data warehouse with an analytic engine, Clinical Looking Glass, which is available to build and analyze de-identified cohorts.

Cohort Definition

Patients were identified and assigned to one of two groups based upon an outpatient prescription with either atorvastatin or simvastatin.

We attempted to build true inception cohorts (first-time use of a specific statin and first-time use of any statin). We used atorvastatin as an example. We demanded that six criteria be met:

- The atorvastatin outpatient prescription would have to be the first outpatient atorvastatin prescription in a patient aged 40 years or older.
- There could be no evidence of any statin prescription in the preceding 10 years.
- The patient would have to have an available LDL and hemoglobin A1c in the year preceding this first atorvastatin prescription.
- There would have to be at least one hemoglobin A1c drawn in the preceding year with a value less than 6.5%.
- Over the preceding two years, there could not be a single hemoglobin A1c value greater than or equal to 6.5%.

This resulted in the selection of a group of patients either provably not diabetic or diabetics under tight control. We applied the same criteria to the simvastatin cohort.

The question we are trying to answer is whether we should prescribe atorvastatin using the life experience of our patient population as a simulation. By somewhat counterintuitively using simvastatin, another statin as a control with presumably similar class effects for the development of diabetes and for the mortality-protective effects of cholesterol-lowering agents, we will bias the study hazard ratio downward toward one for the development of diabetes and death. If simvastatin causes diabetes, then using it as a control for an atorvastatin comparison will attenuate any evaluation difference in diabetic outcome. If patients treated with atorvastatin are found to have a significantly greater likelihood of developing diabetes, then we would infer that an even greater true difference would be seen if the comparison were against a true non diabetes-causing control.

Similarly, if simvastatin protects against death, then any relative risk of death protection shown by our study would be an underestimate of the true death-protective effect of atorvastatin. The technique we are invoking is **bias in service of inference**. We cannot eliminate bias, but we can harness its directionality. By making sure that the bias is against what we want to observe, if we continue to observe a difference and the difference is significant, then the true difference would be even greater.

I have purposely chosen as a control the same class of drug in order to protect against confounding by indication. Doctors often choose to prescribe specific drugs because of their clinical concerns, and this choice may not be equivalent to random assignment. As a result, patients prescribed different drugs are not comparable at baseline to the extent that the doctor's reason for prescribing a particular drug may be indicative of the physician's suspicion of lurking disease. By choosing drugs that are of the same class and are used for the same indications, the possibility of confounding by indication is minimized. Baseline measures in Table 55 and Table 56 will bear out the success of this effort.

Outcome Measure

For each patient, we sought two outcomes—development of diabetes and death.

The case definition for diabetes was evidence of a HgbA1c of $\geq 6.5\%$, the American Diabetes Association threshold for diabetes. Each patient was followed for a maximum of 1,460 days or until they were censored by death or we ran out of follow-up time. The cumulative percent of the cohort developing diabetes was calculated as the complement of the Kaplan-Meier statistic.

Similarly, the cumulative percent who died was calculated using information about death from both the EMRs and death data obtained from Social Security death tapes. In November 2011, Social Security reduced the sensitivity of its publicly distributed death tapes by 50% by not reporting data obtained from state sources only.

A sensitivity analysis will be performed using two strategies. One strategy will restrict death to death detected in our hospital, ignoring the Social Security registry. The second will use a matching strategy requiring that in the matched sets each atorvastatin patient is matched on inception date with a simvastatin patient within the same year-quarter. This matching will create comparability of sensitivity to death in the Social Security registry across groups.

Duration and Assignment of Exposure

Patients were assigned to a specific statin group based upon first statin prescription in our EMR. While we assess the persistence of use of a specific agent between years 2–3, our analysis uses intention to treat based upon the first prescription. The outcome impact of downstream drug switching or nonadherence biases to the null. Thus, the true difference exceeds any demonstrated difference. Since the practical question is "Should we prescribe atorvastatin?" the real-world downstream behavior of patient compliance and switch reflects the experience of our patients, thereby providing a locally relevant effectiveness measure.

Statistical Analysis

A univariate analysis of the cumulative percent developing diabetes or dying will be displayed with the complement of the Kaplan-Meier survival curve. Incidence density is calculated by dividing the number of events by the sum of observed person years. Incidence density relative risk is then calculated by dividing the incidence density of death in atorvastatin by that in simvastatin. Multivariate analyses include the Cox proportional hazard and risk regression.[67,68]

Matching is performed using both a propensity score with the identified variables as well as a requirement that the individual patient matches must also achieve matches within specified tolerances on each variable.[85] This latter requirement corrects for the failure of the propensity matched method to achieve balance at the individual match level for each specific attribute. The algorithm gives priority to the inclusion of the atorvastatin group with the reuse of simvastatin controls if there is no appropriate new simvastatin control. The reuse of controls is recognized by a match weight included in the model building. The success of the matches was evaluated with routines described by Sekhon.[86]

These advanced statistical modeling procedures were implemented and integrated in R by Scry Health (New Haven, CT) in a package we developed for our own institutional use and soon to be available as a commercial package. Variables considered for inclusion in our model included age; dichotomous race (white/not white); dichotomous ethnicity (Hispanic/not Hispanic); gender; last hemoglobin A1c, BMI, and LDL in the year prior to the start of statin; and specific statin. Medical severity scores were developed with a modification of the Charlson Comorbidity Index[43,44,46] based upon all inpatient, outpatient, and emergency department diagnoses available from care delivered at Montefiore in the year preceding the outpatient statin prescription. A second model teased out components of the Charlson for model inclusion: congestive heart failure, myocardial infarction, cerebrovascular disease, and diabetes (none, uncomplicated, complicated). These variables were retained in our models when they achieved a nominal significance of .05 for retention using a backward elimination approach.

Cox proportional hazard ratios are provided as are the 95% confidence intervals. The pure proportionality assumption is easily violated by standard statistical significance criteria in large datasets and is ignored.[87,88] We expect that the model is provably imperfect and provably not purely proportional but that the signal component from the proportionality model is valuable, especially in light of the noncrossover of the Kaplan-Meier plot.

To confirm that the proportionality violating Cox model was still providing meaningful inference, we undertook matched risk regression where one of the matching variables was the exact year and quarter of cohort member enrollment. By forcing the creation of matched synthetic sets where the matches matched exactly on the year and quarter of enrollment, we assured that each matched pair had equal time to manifest the outcome and that the time period of exposure had the same meaningfulness in terms of sensitivity for the detection of the outcome and that they benefitted equally from global changes in practice in secular time.

Data Collection
All patients cared for in the Montefiore Medical Center and its outpatient facilities have their clinical data (laboratory tests, clinical findings, clinical encounters, radiology reports, pathology reports, and prescriptions) recorded in an EMR. The data from this medical record is replicated in a clinical data warehouse used by Clinical Looking Glass,[89] an advanced cohort-building application, to create cohorts and follow them to outcomes in the restricted mode without the need for accessing patient identity. The use of this clinical data for quality improvement and clinical operations is permitted by our internal HIPAA oversight process through a special committee, the Decision Support Group.

Research when undertaken using this tool is reviewed and approved by the Institutional Review Board. Quality improvement and operational analyses to improve or inform care does not require IRB review when the analysis is retrospective.

The entire analysis described in this study was performed without revealing patient identifiers and was undertaken as part of ongoing surveillance of the relevance of findings in the medical literature to our population health interventions in the Bronx. This study was approved by the Institutional Review Board of the Albert Einstein College of Medicine protocol #2014–3985.

Neighborhood socioeconomic status is calculated with the method of Diez Roux[12] using a home address mapped to US Census data and presented as standard deviation units from the New York State mean.

Results

From January 1, 2005, through January 1, 2014, 11,233 patients were found eligible for cohort inclusion. Figure 66 demonstrates the number of patients enrolled by year and quarter in atorvastatin and simvastatin groups.

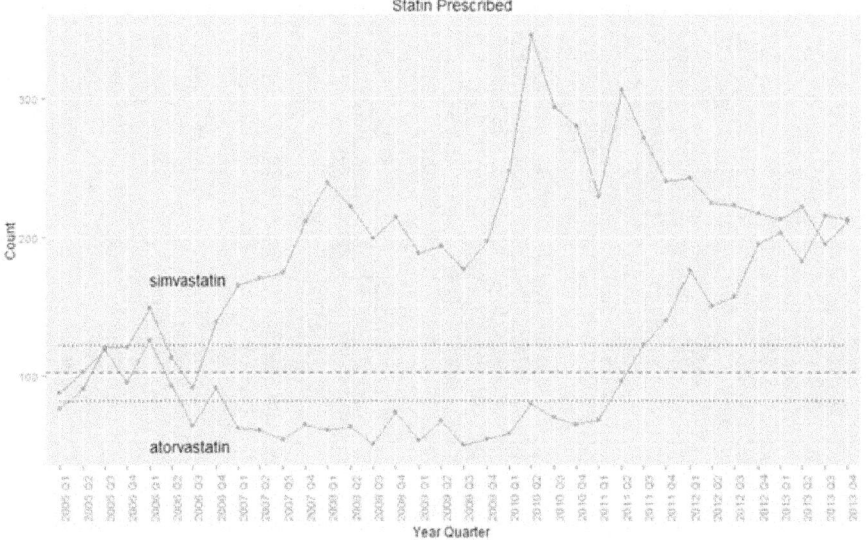

Figure 66. Patient enrollment by year and quarter

Demographic continuous variables are summarized in Table 55, and categorical variables are summarized in Table 56, demonstrating baseline comparability of the two groups.

Table 55. Continuous baseline variables in atorvastatin and simvastatin cohorts

Age (Percentiles)	Atorvastatin	Simvastatin
10th	46	48
25th	52	54
50th	61	63
75th	71	73
90th	79	82
HgbA1c (Percentiles)		
10th	5.2	5.2
25th	5.5	5.4
50th	5.7	5.7
75th	6.0	6.0
90th	6.2	6.2
LDL (Percentiles)		
10th	68	63
25th	93	87
50th	128	120
75th	159	151
90th	187	178
BMI (Percentiles)*		
10th	22.4	22.1
25th	25.4	25.2
50th	28.9	28.8
75th	33.5	33.1
90th	38.7	38.7
Charlson Comorbidity (Percentiles)		
10th	1	1
25th	1	2
50th	3	3
75th	4	4
90th	6	6
SES neighborhood** (sd from New York State Mean)		
10th	-7.35	-7.27
25th	-5.85	-5.78
50th	-2.39	-2.39
75th	-.84	-.95
90th	.44	.11

*Only 6,093 have a BMI record

Table 56. Categoric baseline variables in atorvastatin and simvastatin cohorts

	Atorvastatin	Simvastatin
Number	3,798	7,425
Gender	1,692 (45%)	3,394 (46%)
Ethnicity Hispanic	1,433 (38%)	2,898 (39%)
Race Not White	3,028 (80%)	5,929 (80%)
Cerebrovascular Disease	454 (12%)	1,163 (15.7%)
Congestive Heart Failure	293 (7.7%)	797 (10.7%)
Myocardial Infarction	236 (6.2%)	541 (7.3%)
Peripheral Vascular Disease	168 (4.4%)	363 (4.9%)
Diabetes* **None** **Without Complications** **With Complications**	2,975 (78%) 677 (17.8%) 146 (3.8%)	5,902 (79.4%) 1,200 (16.2%) 323 (4.4%)

*Diabetes diagnosis provided at least once in the year prior to medication prescription.

All diagnoses are based upon the application of the Charlson criteria to diagnoses available from inpatient, outpatient, and emergency department diagnoses in the year prior to prescription.

Patients treated with atorvastatin crossed the ADA HgbA1c threshold of 6.5% more quickly than did the simvastatin group (P=.007) (Figure 68).

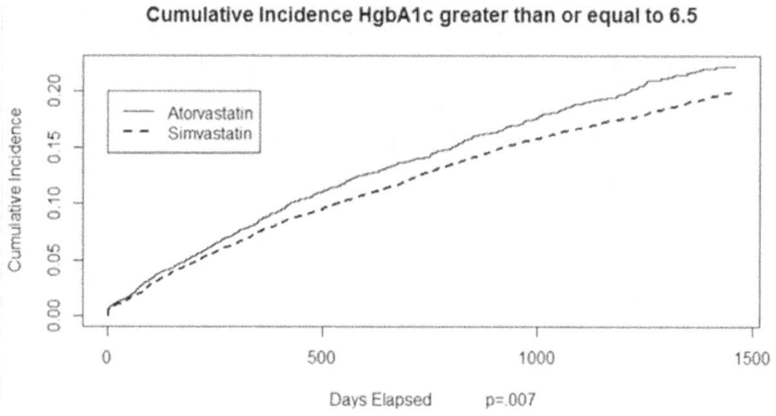

Cumulative Incidence HgbA1c greater than or equal to 6.5

Figure 67. Cumulative percent who achieve a HgbA1c greater than or equal to 6.5%

By 1,460 days (4 years), 22.2% of the atorvastatin crossed the threshold compared with 20.0% of the simvastatin group (Figure 68). The Relative Risk by Incidence Density Method is 1.15 (1.04,1.26).

Using the Cox proportional hazard model, the atorvastatin hazard ratio for the ADA diabetic threshold cross was 1.11 (1.01,1.23), controlling for a history of diabetes in the preceding year, baseline hemoglobin A1c, age, and race (Table 57).

Table 57. Hazard ratio Cox proportional hazard models for variables predictive of HgbA1c≥6.5%

Variable	Hazard Ratio	P value
Atorvastatin vs. simvastatin	1.11 (1.01,1.23)	.03
Race: not white vs. white	1.41 (1.23,1.61)	8 e -7
Age	0.995 (0.991,0.999)	.012
HgbA1c (latest in year previous to statin)	5.37 (4.65,6.21)	<2 e -16
Diabetes without complications*	4.13 (3.73,4.57)	2 e -16
Diabetes with complications*	5.67 (4.85,6.63)	2 e -11

*Baseline—no diabetes diagnosis in the preceding year

Gender and ethnicity (Hispanic/not Hispanic) were not significant predictors. The relative risk regression ignoring exposure time continued to demonstrate significance of atorvastatin (p=.046).

Of the 11,233 patients, 823 died.

Simvastatin patients died at a faster rate than did atorvastatin patients.

Cumulative percent dead in 1,460 days in the simvastatin group was 9.8% compared with atorvastatin at 6.6% (Figure 70) (P=3 e -8). The relative risk incidence density of atorvastatin vs simvastatin was 0.65 (.55, .76). Ignoring Social Security death data and repeating the analysis restricted to deaths detected only on the inpatient service of Montefiore continued to show statistically significant protection by atorvastatin (p=.006).

Using Cox proportional hazard modeling, atorvastatin was protective against death .77 (.65, .90).

Death

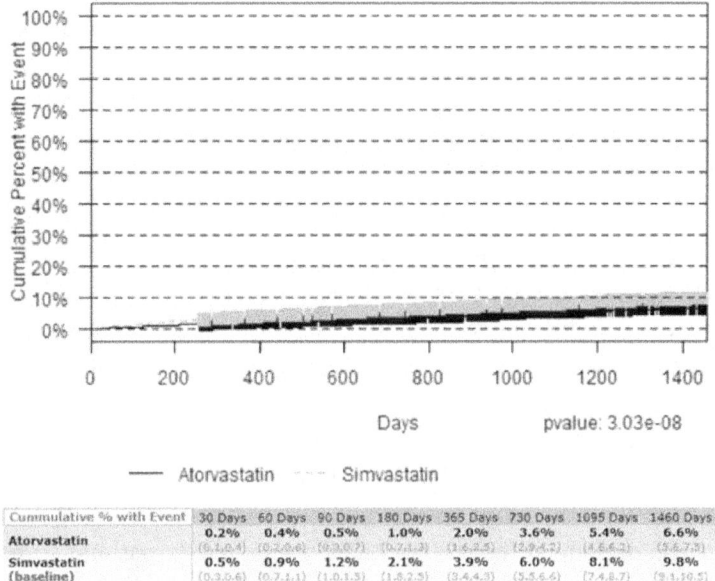

Cummulative % with Event	30 Days	60 Days	90 Days	180 Days	365 Days	730 Days	1095 Days	1460 Days
Atorvastatin	0.2%	0.4%	0.5%	1.0%	2.0%	3.6%	5.4%	6.6%
	(0.1,0.4)	(0.2,0.6)	(0.3,0.7)	(0.7,1.3)	(1.6,2.5)	(2.9,4.2)	(4.6,6.2)	(5.6,7.5)
Simvastatin (baseline)	0.5%	0.9%	1.2%	2.1%	3.9%	6.0%	8.1%	9.8%
	(0.3,0.6)	(0.7,1.1)	(1.0,1.5)	(1.8,2.5)	(3.4,4.3)	(5.5,6.6)	(7.4,8.7)	(9.1,10.5)

Figure 69. Cumulative percent who died

Table 58. Hazard ratios for variables predictive of death

Variables	Hazard Ratio	P value
Atorvastatin vs. simvastatin	0.77 (0.65,0.90)	.001
Male vs. female	1.16 (1.01,1.35)	.04
Age	1.06 (1.05,1.06)	2 e -16
Hispanic vs. not Hispanic	0.74 (0.62,0.87)	.0003
HgbA1c (last in year preprescription)	0.8 (0.68,0.95)	.0099
LDL (last in the year preprescription)	0.993 (0.991,0.995)	2.7 e -11
Diabetes no complications*	1.24 (1.04,1.49)	.02
Diabetes with complications*	1.70 (1.31,2.19)	5 e -5
Congestive heart failure	2.37 (2.00,2.80)	2 e -16
Cerebrovascular disease	1.33 (1.12,1.57)	.002

Race not significant
*Baseline diabetes not diagnosed in the preceding year

Rising hemoglobin A1c was protective against death 0.8 (0.68,0.95)(p=.01). Creating matched synthetic subsets matching atorvastatin and simvastatin on year-quarter and building a multivariable Cox model, including the same variables as the parent data set, continued to show atorvastatin protective 0.77 (0.62,.94) (p=.002).

The presence of at least one same-statin prescription in between day 730 to day 1,095 was 21.8% (20.1%, 23.5%) for atorvastatin and 19.6% (18.5%,20.6%) for simvastatin. Evidence of the use of the comparator statin between days 730 and 1,095 differing from that first prescribed was 5.8% (5.2%,6.4%) for those initiated on atorvastatin and 12.7% (11.4%,14.1%) for those initiated on simvastatin. Inconsistency in medication assignment would bias to the null.

Evidence of a continuing relationship with our health care delivery system was estimated through evidence of at least one office visit or at least one laboratory test between days 730 and 1,460.

The outpatient visit criteria demonstrated that continuity of care in the atorvastatin group was 77% (75.1%,73.7%) and in the simvastatin group was 69.8% (68.5%,71.0%). The laboratory test criteria demonstrated continuity of care in the atorvastatin group to be 75.2% (73.3%,77.0%) and simvastatin to be 68.8% (67.5%,70%).

Discussion

The current analysis clearly demonstrates the propensity of patients treated with atorvastatin to cross the ADA diabetic threshold of HgbA1c≥6.5 significantly faster than simvastatin. If we believe that simvastatin itself can cause diabetes, then this increase over the simvastatin baseline further confirms the diabetogenic effect of atorvastatin. The baseline variables are remarkably similar, and further modeling and matching continues to show this effect. By choosing as a control group another statin, I have reduced confounding by indication as both atorvastatin and simvastatin are given for similar clinical indications and suspicion. The baseline variable similarities bear out this assertion.

Increased baseline HgbA1c is associated with a higher likelihood of crossing the threshold as would seem to be logical. Older age seems to be protective against increasing diabetes. This paradox may be explained by the design of the cohort that guaranteed at least two years of either good control or no diabetes. If your baseline age was older and you still had not yet developed diabetes, then it is more likely that you will not develop diabetes later.

Our style of using bias in the service of inference is especially powerful in our mortality analysis. If we believe that simvastatin is protective against death, then using it as the control group and still demonstrating that atorvastatin is protective against death compared with simvastatin suggests that atorvastatin would be even more impressive were it compared to a nonactive control.

The mortality-protective effect of elevated HgbA1c at baseline .80 (.68,.95) would be more surprising were it not for the results of the Accord study.[90,91] The Accord study showed us that tight HgbA1c control was associated with higher mortality. Since all the diabetic patients in this study were well controlled (<6.5%), those on the tighter spectrum and lower baseline HgbA1c would have been predicted by Accord to have a higher risk of death. Whether the protection against death that we are seeing in our study is due to the HgbA1c elevation (less good control of diabetes), protecting the patient against our overzealous efforts to control blood glucose, or whether the increased survival is due to the more potent effects of the atorvastatin in lowering cholesterol is unclear. What is clear is that in our population the choice to treat with atorvastatin is associated with a lower mortality rate.

The current study used an intention to treat analysis (ITT). This approach is familiar to the aficionados of the randomized controlled trial where intervention assignment for the purpose of analysis is locked at the time of randomization. The purpose of the ITT analysis is to protect the inferential legitimacy of the randomization with its defense against bias at the expense of the power of the study to demonstrate a difference.

In this study, the ITT approach is protecting the initial therapeutic decision at which time, by modeling or matching, I have balanced the effects of covariates at first prescription. We are evaluating the impact of this decision through a functional simulation using the data in the EMR to show the downstream consequences of that initial decision on the death and development of ADA-significant hemoglobin A1c levels ≥6.5 as practiced. Evidence of actual prescription persistence by at least one prescription of the original statin in the third year of follow-up was low in both groups, atorvastatin (21.8%) and simvastatin (18.5%). That we continued to find largely significant differences in both analytic outcomes, despite the poor adherence and therefore functional misclassification of true therapy, suggests that the interventions are even more potent than reported. We relied on evidence of prescriptions in the EMR to substantiate ongoing use. Discussion with some practitioners reveals that some did not record renewals in the system, so the actual prevalence of renewed medication is unknown.

Some may find the use of the language of the randomized controlled trial (RCT) in what is clearly not an RCT somewhat cheeky. I would argue that what is at stake here is a classic argument between efficacy and effectiveness. Efficacy asks whether the drug works when tested in a controlled trial with willing subjects and tight inclusion and exclusion criteria. Effectiveness asks whether the drug works when used in practice with the vagaries of human behaviors of both doctors and patients once an initial assignment has been made.

It is this latter question of effectiveness that our style of analysis is addressing. We found patients from the time of their first outpatient prescription with simvastatin or atorvastatin and made sure that they were on no other statin before. The effectiveness question seeks to determine the natural history of the patients whose initial chosen statin was simvastatin or atorvastatin. We tried to adjust for the relevant variables at decision time to make sure we had comparability at this baseline decision and then tracked outcomes.

Death evaluation was challenged by the changing sensitivity of the Social Security death tapes. By repeating the analysis, matching the two cohorts on inception date within year-quarter, we forced equal potential time of exposure to the changing death sensitivity. This approach also forced equal exposure to temporal changes in other therapies that might have confounded the outcome.

Standard analyses use modeling to extract inference on the significance of the explanatory variables. Modeling, by its very nature, adds assumptions in order to draw analytic strength from data in cohort members who do not exactly match members in the other group in their covariates but can testify as to the impact of their variable values on the observed outcome. Such assumptions can be somewhat hidden but include such things as normal errors or linear relationships.

By contrast, matching, as an analytic strategy, makes fewer assumptions and is intrinsically more transparent. We require that each member of one group has a matched pair in the other group where all the appropriate variables are matched within certain tolerances so that the only relevant difference is group membership. The cost of this transparency and smaller number of assumptions is the elimination of those who do not have a match with a resultant loss of analytic power. The more variables you try to match, the fewer resultant people will survive the matching process to form the synthetic matched sets.

In our mortality analysis, we used the best of both worlds in a reasonable compromise. We forced a match on year-quarter for the date of first medication. This reduced the primary threat to external validity caused by the changing sensitivity in our Social Security death measure. But we reserved the other adjustments with previously determined significant variables to be handled by Cox multivariable analysis on the synthetic matched sets, thereby drawing strength from similar by not exactly matched patients.

Limitations

As in all observational studies, there are potential limitations. We created our cohorts so they would be composed of patients with a known first date of statin use. While we had access to a powerful information system, we cannot eliminate the possibility that a patient was actually started on a statin in another health care delivery system.

Table 55 demonstrates 10% of the patients in both simvastatin and atorvastatin groups with LDL levels so low as to be suggestive of treatment by statin within the year preceding our first evidence of outpatient prescription. Fortunately, the actual breakdown of values in LDL does not show a dramatic difference in the proportions between the two groups.

We cannot eliminate the possibility of unmeasured confounders, but the fact that the indications for both drugs are similar should have at least attenuated, if not eliminated, the issue of confounding by indication.

BMI was only present in 53% of our patients as, in the early years, BMI was not reliably recorded in the outpatient record. As a result, we could not use BMI in our models without a serious loss of patient number and statistical power.

Evidence of continuity of care in our system using outpatient visits was 77% for atorvastatin and 69.8% for simvastatin. We would have liked to have evidence of complete follow-up with information from hospitals in our vicinity such as will ultimately be possible from regional health information organizations. The present incompleteness may be a source of potential confounding.

A recent blog review of big data medical claims by William Hersh[92] properly identified that the exuberant promises made for clinical and public policy utility exceeded the published evidence. This study is a clear example of how a focused clinical question attempting to confirm a hypothesis and then explore a consequence can yield guidance from a big data repository.

Dr. Hersh is undoubtedly correct that the hype exceeds the reality for the moment. To undertake big data analysis in medicine, one needs four items: two tools, a trained operator, and a focused question.

The first tool is a cohort builder—a system that allows you to assemble patients with specific characteristics at their time of inclusion (index date) as well as characteristics within specified time frames of this index date.[3,89] The cohort builder should be able to assemble relevant data on the included members of the cohort for univariate and multivariate analyses.

A second set of tools must permit advanced analytics with modeling, matching, and the ability to analyze time to multiple events with matched subsets.

The last two components are an epidemiologically aware operator who understands the biases of his data sets creation and a focused clinical question or hypothesis. With these four components, we can begin to expect that additional work like that described herein will convert the EMR from a glorified file cabinet into a source of care guidance.

Conclusion

Atorvastatin is associated with diabetes onset, but in our population, the net effect of prescribing atorvastatin is protective against death. Big data analytics using local EMR data can contextualize through functional simulation the implications of specific clinical decisions made in practice as the downstream patient and clinician decisions play out in practice—a true effectiveness metric. Such observations should become more frequent as tools, data, and skills proliferate with the hope that they will guide therapy and policy.

Machine Learning and Surveillance: Help, Hype, or Both?

Extracting inference from electronic medical data is a huge and complex undertaking, way beyond a simple single-chapter summary.[93-101] However, I have included this section to warn about a dangerous creeping attitude with a tendency to delay or obscure meaningful discussion about realizable goals.

One can think of three categories of learning: standard statistical modeling, machine learning, and deep machine learning.

Old-school statistical models using imperfect models were able to extract meaning from complex clinical observation. The meaning extracted were of two types: prediction of outcome for a population or inference with determination of the impact of a specific causal variable (treatment or risk factor).

Good predictive models permit targeting the subpopulation at the highest risk of adverse outcomes, thus efficiently using scarce resources to get the most bang for the buck.

Identifying a causal agent, be it effective treatment or a specific risk factor, permit planning and implementing an intervention that targets the cause and is preventive of negative outcomes.

For these models to work in days past,[45,102] the operator needed to identify the variables of interest and their functional form. Is age important? Is age important as a linear trend? As a factor with three levels: 40–65, 65–75, and 75–85? Is a higher order of age important—square or to the third power? Should we force the values of the variable to assume a more normal distribution by using a log transform?

What compromises are you willing to make in understandability of the model and its coefficients as related to real-world items of interest (odds ratios, relative risk, risk difference) in order to obtain greater accuracy in prediction and better calibration of the model over the range of values?

In addition to these statistical modeling questions, there were questions of variable meaning. Which drug classes have meaning? Do we look at each drug by itself, or do we collapse all the drugs of a common type—say, antidepressants, or more narrowly, antidepressants that work as selective serotonin reuptake inhibitors? We map these concepts into dummy variables whose values are yes or no (1, 0). How do we recognize drug adherence before we count a drug as present? Does the patient have to be adherent from a refill perspective more than 50% of the time? How do we represent adherence in a model when the cause of the non-adherence may be side effects, which should be considered before instituting an intervention with the drug?

As you can see, the clinical, methodological, and statistical thought required can be complex and can benefit from the experience of the study designer, but it is also visibly subject to the limitations of his skill and subjective choices.

Machine learning can run through many statistical models and functional forms of the variables, evaluate the relative quality of those models, and choose between them through internal performance checks with cross-validation. We can allow multiple models and forms to behave in ensembles voting for the appropriate prediction (random forest) and impose a weighting algorithm on the individual model's vote based upon past prediction success. Even in machine learning, the human experience of the functional forms of the outcome, the explanatory variables, and the creation of the variables themselves are prerequisites for building useful predictive and explanatory models.

Deep learning holds out the promise of a free lunch. Presumably, you do not need to think. You do not need experience. All you have to do is point the machine at a huge number of observations and variables, and the machine will learn with its built-in default settings for loss and unimpeachable criteria for model superiority. Without going into the details, we have seen amazing results in image recognition and language translation.

Many nonspecialists have misunderstood this as an implicit promise that we do not need to know much or think much but that we must simply hire the right machine team and intone the magical incantation "artificial intelligence" (AI), and all will be solved. For administrative leaders whose skill set has deteriorated to choosing between two consultant-vetted options, this further avoidance of difficult thought is too enticing an offer to resist.

It has a black-box quality. We do not know what it is really doing, but it must be powerful because it has demonstrated that power already. It now derives legitimacy from performance in other domains with profoundly different structural assumptions and intellectual challenges. Images, for example, are made up of pixels with differing intensities and spatial relations. The pixel, however, is an unambiguous finding (x,y Cartesian position: 54,67, intensity strong). The outcome ("this is a cat") is knowable with reasonable certainty, and the training material capturing the domain is nearly infinite in the universe that Google ingests.

Translation also benefits from an unlimited supply of training material with unambiguous substrate (the word in the foreign language) and the unambiguous outcome (the word in the target language). I am slightly overstating it as there are inherent circularities and ambiguities in human language, but the substrate and outcome have a stability and clarity often missing in the clinical arena.

Ongoing success depends upon the static maintenance of the stability of the environment in which it was trained. This is not different from previous modeling efforts. However, while all models can deteriorate over time in unanticipated ways, the black-box failure to focus us on potential variables of dependent weakness and our undue reverence causing us to foreswear explicit ongoing performance surveillance put us at greater risk.

Google scientists[103] ran an experiment relying upon such a promise in health care and applied enormous computing resources to the EMRs of two major hospitals. The team purposely did not employ any human preprocessing of data elements. It did not standardize medications by categories or standardize language but allowed the entirety of the notes of the medical record to be ingested and turned into a huge number of variables without any human clinical guidance.

No concept of laboratory value badness.

No concept of category of drug (anxiolytic, antidepressant).

No concept of certainty of finding.

The machine was asked to use its raw substrate to drive a predictive model that would predict death during the hospital stay. The model was tested at different days of the hospitalization to demonstrate prediction performance on different hospital days. Deeper into the admission, additional information became available, and the people still left to be predicted were reduced by those who had already died. This last point, I am not sure of in my reading of the paper, but it would be an important consideration, as you need to predict with the information available at the time of the prediction about the population available to receive a prediction.

Reported predicted mortality was impressive. However, what is not generally appreciated by the public, although clearly stated in the paper, is the fact that although the model predicted well in each individual hospital, there was no way to use the learning in hospital A to inform hospital B predictions. The idiosyncratic use of language and variable constructs discovered in each but unstandardized by a tedious human activity created independent universes that could not share knowledge between them. The words and phrases did not have the stability that pixels and intensity have in the image classification modeling.

The implication, at the moment, is that you would have to build knowledge locally, and since most individual hospitals do not have a large enough target data, this process would require collecting data over a long enough period of time to create locally meaningful predictions.

The problem, of course, is that not all local systems are able to produce enough data to overcome the idiosyncratic variability of their data substrate to allow for prediction, and as we already saw, without standardization of language (medication, labs, etc.). Also, as you increase the time window, you may be capturing data elements (drugs or procedures) that are no longer in common use and therefore serve as a functional secular time variable rather than as a useful contemporaneous predictor variable.

We should distinguish between machine learning and machine surveillance. Once a model is developed, be it by any of the three categories—standard statistical, machine learning, or deep learning—it can be employed for surveillance on the hospitalized patient population.

I suspect we will find that even the deep machine-learning algorithms will turn out to be hybrid, in the sense that the variables will be human-recognizable variables (respiratory rate, blood pressure, change of recognizable variables over time) that are generalizable between institutions. Without this generalizability, their marketability will be very constrained so that economic drivers, in addition to substantive clinical considerations, will drive the use of clearly recognizable variables whose functional forms are negotiated in the deep layers of the machine-learning algorithms.

The latter, driven by human-recommended variables potentially weighted by machine-learning algorithms, can maintain surveillance of patients whose findings are often ignored in practice by distracted and busy clinicians. Machine surveillance can collect patients' blood pressure, temperature, and respiratory rate and then attempt to identify those patients who are deteriorating and needing aggressive intervention to prevent respiratory arrest or septic shock.

A number of important questions must then be asked.

- How well does the predictive surveillance model perform?
  - In patients who have the disease, what is the sensitivity of the model?
  - For those without the disease, what is the specificity (the complement of the false positive rate)?
  - When the test is applied in the population of interest,
    - How often isthe signal generated actually a true positive (the positive predictive value)?
    - What number of patients must be tested to find one true positive?
    - How often is the lack of a signal evidence of a disease-free status (negative predictive value)?
    - How many of the diseased patients are actually captured by the model (coverage)?
    - How many false signal events are you encountering, and what is their cost in order to get the coverage you have achieved?

These are the standard questions that must be asked of any model of any sophistication. The models must be built on a training set and then validated on a testing set. All elements of the model must be built on the training set—coefficients and threshold values for decision making. The testing set must be tested with the models and their thresholds previously determined from the training set to understand how well the model performs.

Once you have your model in hand, you are not done. You now must ask the following.

- What interventions can be brought to bear?
- How effective are these interventions if done properly?
- How well are these interventions executed in your environment? We will need to maintain surveillance on the execution if we are to continue to benefit.
- What is the measurable impact on the clinical issue of interest?
- What are the opportunity costs on other patients deprived of our clinical concern drained by this activity? The opportunity cost is often the least

considered, but it is important when there are scarce resources, which is always the case.

Using machine surveillance for the precursors of respiratory arrest or septic shock could create signals to interventionist teams to reach those patients to prevent their deterioration.[104] In some cases, it is not the discovery of new variables but rather the enhanced attention of 24x7 continual surveillance of known variables that adds the benefit. In other cases, it is assumed that the confluence of multiple measures in temporal proximity produces a signal otherwise hidden from clinician awareness.

Both of these possibilities are intriguing for the improvement of patient outcome on the factory floor of the modern hospital. Of course, formal evaluation is required, which includes the calculation of sensitivity, specificity, predictive value of a positive, false-positive identification rate in practice, predictive value of a negative, and assessment of impact on hard outcomes.

In assessing these important metrics, it is critical not to confuse the false positive rate—the complement of the specificity derived in a population 100% without the disease with the false positive rate of the signal in the context of real-world use where it has to contend with the nasty reality of the low prevalence of the condition of interest.

An ostensibly impressive predictor of in-hospital death or in-hospital respiratory failure resulting in >48 hours of machine ventilation was built with machine learning.[104] In its prospective validation trial, it reported an impressive area under the ROC (AUROC) curve of .87 and a false positive rate of 5% at its chosen internal cutoff. However, when applied in the population of interest, the positive predictive value was only 16%, meaning that 84% of the time that the alarm went off, the signal was wrong.

Of course, this is a well-understood phenomenon. The utility of the prediction algorithm must take into consideration the prevalence of the outcome condition. Because the outcome condition—death or respiratory failure—is rare, the false positive rate of 5% creates dramatically more false signals as a contributor to all the alarms than can be compensated by those patients generating the true signal.

Positive Predictive Value

$$= \frac{(Sensitivity * Prevalence)}{(Sensitivity * Prevalence) + (1 - Specificity) * (1 - Prevalence)}$$

The impact of prevalence on the positive predictive value is profound.

Let us use as an example data on the approve measure[104] for detecting patients who will either die in 24 hours or who will have respiratory failure requiring at least 48 hours of ventilator support.

Sensitivity=0.64, Specificity=.95

An automated surveillance tool applied to all the patients in the hospital will generate a true signal—a positive predictive value of 11.4% for a prevalence of 1%, 21% for a prevalence of 2%, and 76% for a prevalence of 20%. In the unstated prevalence in the article, we are told of a positive predictive value of 16%, which, through the equation above, implies a prevalence of 1.47%.

The low number of patients who are either going to die or who will require mechanical ventilation for more than 24 hours results in this low positive predictive value.

In addition to these statistical issues, opportunity cost must also be evaluated as resources of staff time are drained from other concerns that are not the focus of this effort. Other patients might therefore pay the price of lost resource and focus. Often this collateral damage is not even considered, with victory declared in the narrow focus of the intervention without truly establishing the larger cost.

Even more frustrating to the proponents of AI-directed interventions might be the possibility (yet to be assessed) that the prevention of the present antecedents to death will only reveal another unrecognized cause hiding in the shadows of the first. These patients suffer from multiple comorbidities, and the removal of one proximate cause of death may only lead to the revelation of the next. It is for this very reason that the careful assessment of interventions, goals, and outcomes is important.

Artificial intelligence is a wonderful tool and undoubtedly will improve our capabilities to detect preventable problems that are currently being ignored. However, we should remember that AI is always best when it is augmented by the neural net located between our ears—human intelligence.

What Do We Need Prediction For?

P rediction has the following components:

- Care delivery utility—to target people for proactive interventions.
- Quality comparison utility—to permit entities to compare their performance with other institutions by "adjusting for" what would be expected by virtue of predictive variables that differ between institutions.
- Reimbursement utility—to allow risk-bearing care delivery systems to be properly compensated for the complexity of the patients in their care.

Care Delivery Utility

The amount of lead time for predictive models can differ dramatically. The pooled cohort risk assessment equations predict a 10-year risk for a first atherosclerotic cardiovascular disease (ASCVD) event and are used in clinical practice to justify lipid-lowering agents in primary prevention strategies. Lead time is of the order of years to a decade.

Predictive models of the preceding chapter for in-hospital interventions had a lead time of hours.

These use cases are for proactive interventions before the endpoint is reached, although it could be argued that many in-hospital predictions may be more early detection of endpoint prodrome rather than of pure prediction, changing the paradigm from "predict and prevent" to "detect and remediate quickly."

There are other models more reactive in nature, such as those that stratify patients prior to discharge to anticipate those with a high likelihood of readmission. A formal review of frequent fliers—patients with multiple hospitalizations—by a care management team is functionally using the frequent-flyer designation as a predictive stratifier. But even more complex predictive models can be used to focus a care delivery team empowered with special resources (social service, physician home visits, telephonic follow-up).

Early detection with reactive intervention prior to major resource consumption can sometimes trump predictive modeling when the data (dialysis duration, fluid removal, weight change) is not yet operationally available in real time to develop models with adequate sensitivity and specificity. In the next chapter, we rely upon a dialysis patient's neural net to detect fluid overload, to signal the need for extra dialysis, and to provide an opportunity for that signal to reach an action arm of the delivery system to rapidly provide additional dialysis prior to clinical deterioration requiring an admission. In our fascination with predictive modeling, we must not delay or overlook real opportunities for early detection and remediation that can be done today with less sophisticated approaches.

Quality Comparisons

To evaluate the quality of your care, it is often useful to identify other institutions or health care agents who perform similar activities and compare their reported successes with your own. Complicating this comparison are predictive variables known to be in different proportion in the comparison groups. Without correction for the impact of these baseline differences, conclusions about the relative success of the two programs are questionable.

We can often be blinded by the scientific nature of these models and fail to ask some basic questions. Do the variables in the two populations have the same meaning? Does hospital distance measured in miles in a population with access to a car in the American heartland have the same meaning as the same metric in an urban population whose mode of transportation is mass transit (buses and subways) with delays inherent in transfers and not necessarily in point-to-point distance? Only proactive special efforts produce a car service for urban transportation, so distance has a potentially different meaning.

Of great importance is the missing predictor variable. A cardiologist colleague pointed out that he is involved in two registries that are both looking at mortality rates for patients receiving stents for clinical scenarios of varying anatomic complexities. One of the registries also captures the metric of urgency and of the state of the patient at the time of presentation to the catheterization unit. When patients seen are predominantly elective cases, there is a certain mortality and complication rate. But if the patients are predominantly emergent or brought in after a transient death outside of the hospital, the risk for complications is profoundly different. Not recognizing these dramatic contextual differences creates unfair and meaningless comparisons. In his case, the two registries produce contradictory messages.

No statistical model, not even the messianic AI, can correct for the missing causal variable problem.

Reimbursement Utility: Mutually Assured Destruction—The Race to Clinical Irrelevance

Once health care systems assume full financial risk, both the risk-bearing health systems and insurers have an interest in adjusting for the complexity of their patient population. To prevent provider systems from gaming the situation by creaming the population of the less sick, hoping to obtain the same reimbursement gained by broadly accepting a fair representation of population risk, the federal government has created for its Medicare Advantage program a way to assess the density of clinical disease and risk in a population on a regular basis with significant implications for reimbursement.

Risk is billing diagnosis based and drives a hierarchical condition category (HCC) score. At the end of 2018, Medicare provided the insuring entities a summary of patient diagnoses as well as the HCC score based on those diagnoses that will determine the annual reimbursement that will begin in July of 2019.

At the end of 2018, CMS sent a code file to Montefiore listing all those patients in our Medicare Advantage program and the submitted billing codes that will drive their HCC adjuster. We are given a chance to review the medical records of outpatient visits with a clinician or inpatient visits, and if we can find evidence of a doctor-identified and doctor-stated diagnosis not documented in the billing process, we can submit those additional diagnoses and get credit from CMS for our HCC coding adjustment. This is important because starting midyear, the rates paid by CMS will be informed by this new HCC coding. On average, when new codes are found, the resulting HCC coding enhancement results in somewhere between $200 and $400 per person.

There is a perverse quality to the effort. A patient who has been billed for diabetes uncomplicated and separately for kidney disease is worth far less than if he had been billed as "diabetic with complication of kidney disease."

The reality of the patient is not relevant. You could demonstrate both diabetes and kidney disease from laboratory tests (HgbA1c, estimated glomerular filtration rate), but unless the doctor in his note indicated that the patient had diabetes and kidney disease as a complication of the diabetes, the higher reimbursement would be denied.

As this is economic life and death, a dramatic effort must be made by our health care system to recoup at-risk dollars, so this nonclinical expensive process follows:

Method of Review

1. Contract with a natural language processing (NLP) company with a data tunnel into our EMR system.
2. Our EMR has a flag field identifying patients who are part of Medicare Advantage and eligible for the HCC enhancement.
3. The NLP machine asks our EMR for all the outpatient and inpatient doctors' notes. It then goes through all the documents for each patient, identifying potential text with diagnoses that might be important for HCC coding. These diagnoses are then compared to those previously reported in bills to CMS, and these duplicative findings are suppressed. For those diagnoses not suppressed, a message goes to human coders who then review the actual written text and then accept or reject the validity of the signal. The accepted signals and their documentation become a report for CMS. The system is optimized for sensitivity with a false positive rate of 1–4%. We looked at a week of patient charts reviews and found that 258/4,624 positive alerts were verified as true positives (positive predictive value of 5.6%).
4. For estimated productivity, 32 flagged charts can be processed by coders a day. With five coders and five days a week, this process should reach 800 charts. In the week of our analysis, we found only 237 patients processed, of which 125 (53%) had new diagnoses relevant to the HCC process. Since we had anticipated 800 charts to be reviewed, this low productivity was then explained by not having all five coders due to illness. The NLP software dramatically speeds up the review, both by eliminating any energy spent on

diagnoses already known to CMS and by focusing attention on the relevant text directly. While 32 charts a day can be processed by those who use the NLP program, productivity is much lower in those without the NLP tool. With complicated records and thick inpatient charts, productivity can be as little as 4 a day.

5. High sensitivity at the expense of specificity is critical for financial success and precludes the use of this tool with its present cutoffs for sensitivity and specificity without coder review for general epidemiologic or quality studies. The reason this financial process can tolerate this poor specificity is the fact that the coders find grounds for codes that will result in HCC upcoding in 53% of the charts reviewed. In a back-of-the-envelope calculation, if 32 charts are reviewed because of the NLP signal, 53% are indeed positive, and the range of reimbursement is a $200–400 increase. This means that, at the lower limit, 32*0.53*200, or $3,392 dollars, are being recovered each day per person. A month has 20 days, so in a month $67,840 is retrieved. Since the software license costs $24,000, and since we have five coders, this would come to $4 million.

CMS is working hard to change the rules and prohibit this second bite at the reimbursement apple. They are working to create contracts where you only get credit for what you record at the time of care without permitting a lookback re-documentation process. Doctors do not record as coders might like. While they might acknowledge type 2 diabetes and, somewhere in their note, acknowledge end-stage renal disease, they may not include in their official billing a diagnosis of "type 2 diabetes complicated by end stage renal disease." Since they do not record it as a billing code, CMS does not recognize this fact until the after-the-fact lookback process that we have described.

Our NLP software is limited by the chosen thresholds for sensitivity and specificity. It is presently weighted to sensitivity, so an "alcohol pad" would be flagged as possible PAD (peripheral artery disease), which is then rejected by the coders. Our NLP software is also limited by its limited substrate of data (medical records) upon which it has been trained. With greater experience and a greater number of records, the inherent machine learning will improve.

There are two reporting formats:

- RAPS file with three fields: HIC #, date of service, diagnosis code (no need to include the provider).

- EDPS file with 38 fields, including relevant provider, provider national identifier NPI, etc.

The EDPS file is much more comprehensive and much more error-prone. A single period misplaced in a name or incomplete name with a middle initial can cause a rejection. The federal government wants more of the form submissions to be of the EDPS variety ostensibly because the required physician provider field allows for an audit of both the diagnosis and the physician. The audits are way behind. It is now May 21, 2019, and I was told that the audits have not been done beyond 2014.

Because EDPS files are subject to a higher proportion of rejection for failure in completion, there is a financial advantage for the federal government to require an ever-increasing percentage of the reporting with EDPS files so as to reject claims and not pay them. The health care industry has a hard time countering the rejections, spending large sums of money and technology while being unable to find exactly why the rejection occurred.

The EDPS:RAPS file ratio of reporting is thus a clever bureaucratic way to reduce payouts (and hence cost). The ratio was 15–85, and it is now 25–75. Soon CMS will require 50:50, further worsening the situation.

As you can see, in this coding submission process, we have a situation similar to that between the United States and the USSR in the 1960s and 1970s when both threatened the other with atomic mutually assured destruction (MAD) as a deterrent to atomic war initiation. In the billing wars, CMS and the providers are in an escalating battle, consuming progressively greater resources to deny payment or garner payment, respectively, as provider organizations invest in clinically irrelevant activity at the expense of other more clinically valuable activity.

This energy and attention suck will not stop here as a post clinical encounter process. As of this writing, vendors are proposing systems directly integrated in the EMR to read the physicians' notes and advise physicians in real time to consider more appropriate—i.e., more remunerative—coding. The physician's attention span is already taxed for clinically relevant interventions, and now we will steal more of the physician's time and attention to respond to a system generating false positives and distracting signals. It is a race from value to clinical irrelevance, perversely opposed to the value proposition espoused by CMS.

Observed vs. True Cost Savings: Why Health Systems Do Not Evolve

Background

I f improved quality can generate cost savings, then why do we not see a rapid evolution of health systems to greater quality and savings?

Value enhancement in both clinical outcome and cost savings have not been found with standard activities like JCAHO accreditation.[105] The achievement of better-quality-care metrics has failed to reduce readmission rates after myocardial infarction or heart failure.[106,107] Intensive outpatient program efforts in high-need patients have failed to reduce acute care utilization.[108]

Many resist the painful cognitive dissonance caused by these papers, faulting the particular study's implementation or quality target. Most believe that there must be a way to save money by investing in quality, with some advocating the routine use of the machinery of the randomized control trial to identify those interventions that can deliver the goods.[109]

In this chapter, we present a dialysis patient cost simulation undertaken to anticipate intervention cost savings to justify intervention expenditures. In the course of the work, we began to note a profound difference between true savings predicted by our model and observable savings using control groups—either in the randomized controlled trial or by its poorer cousin but medical chief executive officer (CEO) respected—the observed year-to-year cost comparison.

Our observations explain why, on a local level, over relevant annual budgetary time windows, there may be a lack of positive feedback signals to properly encourage the support of effective interventions. This is a fundamental property of statistics, and it plagues many such efforts leading to premature termination of truly successful interventions or an unwillingness to even initiate them because their success is temporarily invisible. Latency of detectable savings defeats the better impulses of impatient clinical system CEOs, causing them to undervalue performance improvement efforts.

Population

Eligible patients were those age 18 or older for whom the Montefiore Care Management Organization was at full financial risk for all health care, who had been seen at least once in one of Montefiore's inpatient or outpatient facilities, were on dialysis in 2016 (prevalent and incident), and in 365 days after first dialysis in that year had not received a kidney transplant. Patients who died in the year of follow-up were included. Acute care hospital costs were collected in the one year following the first 2016 dialysis.

A hospital admission was deemed "preventable" by our renal specialist if its primary diagnosis was suggestive of inadequate dialysis with fluid overload or electrolyte imbalance, infection, or dialysis access dysfunction.[110,111]

We believed that we could design an intervention to enable timelier patient-initiated access to dialysis, antibiotic therapy, or shunt clearance to prevent these admissions.

Each patient's address is geocoded to census block with neighborhood socioeconomic status (SES) calculated using the method of Roux.[12] The neighborhood SES variable is presented as the number of standard deviations from the mean SES of NY State census blocks.

Population Details

1,394 dialysis patients' demographics are summarized in Table 59.

Table 59. Patient description

Population	N= 1,394
Age	
Mean (std dev)	63.3 (14.11)
Age Percentiles:	$(5^{th}, 25^{th}, 50^{th}, 75^{th}, 95^{th})$
	(37, 44, 54, 73, 81)
Males	737 (53%)
Race	
Black	645 (46%)
Multiple	104 (8%)
Other	389 (28%)
Unknown	123 (9%)
White	133 (10%)
Ethnicity	
Hispanic	336 (24%)
Not Hispanic	779 (56%)
Unknown	279 (20%)
Language (Primary)	
English	1,087 (78%)
Spanish	157 (11%)
Other	25 (2%)
Unknown	125 (9%)
Neighborhood Socioeconomic Status	Percentile
(# of standard deviations from NYS mean)	$(5^{th}, 10^{th}, 25^{th}, 50^{th}, 75^{th}, 90^{th}, 95^{th})$ -8, -7, -6, -2, -1, 0.2, 1

Summarizing hospitalizations and cost in this cohort in 365 days of follow-up from first 2016 dialysis, we find the following:

- 899 (64%) patients with at least one admission during one year of follow-up.
  - 495 (36%) without any admission
- 2,456 admissions
  - Hospital costs: $52,988,472
- 382 (22%) people with at least one "preventable" admission
  - 593 (18.4%) "preventable" admissions
  - Cost of "preventable" admissions: $10,949,878

Statistical Simulations

We simulated true savings variability assuming a 50% effective intervention for the preventable admissions using the following approach.

True Savings Simulation

- Randomly select a sample size of 250 patients with replacement from the original N=1,394 to create a sample of size of 250 representative subjects. Every subject is equally likely to be picked unweighted by the number of admissions or the prior selection. A subject may be selected more than once in the random sampling.
- For those subjects selected, collect all their admissions in the 365 days following the first recorded dialysis in 2016.
- Sum the actual costs of those admissions as experienced.
- For the admissions deemed preventable, assume that 50% of those admissions could have been eliminated with their accompanying costs saved through the proposed intervention. This is accomplished by creating a probabilistic attenuator that eliminates the cost for the preventable admission 50% of the time through a random number generator,[112] R version 3.4.2 (2017-09-28).
- Sum the costs if the intervention was provided with 50% effectiveness.
- Calculate the difference between cost as experienced without treatment minus cost with treatment attenuation. If positive, this is true cost savings.

- Repeat this procedure 5,000 times to create 5,000 universes of savings.
- Sort order using the savings.
- Calculate the percentiles.

To understand a percentile table, consider the 2.5th percentile value.

The amount saved at the 2.5th percentile is the amount saved greater than the first 2.5% of the sort-ordered simulated samples. This means that 97.5% of the simulated samples have a cost saving greater than that seen at the 2.5th percentile. For our purposes, I will call the 2.5th percentile the minimum savings.

The 50th percentile represents the median saved.

The reader is reminded that random resampling in an absolute sense is impossible using computer algorithms. A computer is a deterministic machine that uses a seed start value to algorithmically generate random selection. The same seed generates the same random pattern. Table 60 demonstrates how different row seeds produce different observed percentiles when resampling groups of 250 subjects 5,000 times each.

Table 60. Simulated true savings per person (percentiles) †

	Percentile										
Seed	2.5%	5%	10%	20%	21%	22%	25%	50%	75%	90%	95%
1	**2,583**	2,777	3,015	3,326	3,353	3,371	3,444	3,958	4,521	5,088	5,484
2	2,375	2,544	2,764	3,045	3,073	3,096	3,170	3,619	4,074	4,564	4,874
3	2,620	2,826	3,080	3,395	3,418	3,437	3,513	4,022	4,588	5,127	5,509
4	2,597	2,782	3,007	3,310	3,333	3,355	3,422	3,892	4,406	4,921	5,235
5	2,298	2,458	2,670	2,953	2,975	2,998	3,065	3,529	4,089	4,593	4,933
6	2,570	2,766	2,995	3,308	3,333	3,360	3,433	3,932	4,480	5,017	5,340

† Assumes 50% effectiveness of the intervention on the preventable admissions (six seeds, N=250, 5,000 trials).

In the first row, (seed #1), the 2.5th percentile displays a savings of $2,583 per person, meaning that 97.5% of the time, our intervention with an effectiveness of 50% applied to 250 randomly selected dialysis patients would save at least $2,583 per person by preventing preventable admissions.

In the second row (seed #2), the amount saved per person is minimally only $2,375.

To obtain a reasonable summary estimate, you can run 100 seeds and average the values at each percentile. This is functionally akin to a simulation resampling

500,000 samples of 250 patients each. It will be this larger simulation equivalent that will be used to describe the phenomena of this chapter.

A few important observations. The average of the 2.5th percentiles, which I have called the minimum money saved for groups of sizes of 250 members, is $2,522 per person or $630,500 for the group. The average of the median money saved per person is $3,865 or $966,250 for the group. Increasing the sample size to the entire dialysis population of 1,394 provides a minimum and median per-person savings of $3,289 and $3,909 and group savings of $4,584,866 and $5,449,146, respectively.

As you can see, as the sample size increases, the minimum value approaches the median. The distribution of the cost saving estimates is narrowed. From a CEO perspective, enrolling a larger sample size in the intervention not only increases the number of opportunities to save money by increasing the number of patients treated, but it also obtains a 30% (3,289/2,522) increase in minimum per-person savings.

Note also how the median savings of the 250-member group is 99% (3,865/3,909) of the median savings of the 1,394 group. The median is a pretty stable estimate across sample sizes.

If you apply the $3,909 median savings to the 1,394 patients, you calculate an overall savings of $5,449,146. This is 49.8% of the $10,949,878 savings that we calculated as preventable admission costs in the original cohort and, not surprisingly, close to our model's designed 50% effectiveness. The average of the median values is pretty representative of the true savings.

The assumptions of the aforementioned true cost-savings simulation should now be made explicit as they are striking and will soon make the point that they are only observable in the "eyes of G-d."

In the true cost simulation, we compare the costs between two groups with and without a 50% effective intervention.

However, unrealistically, both the intervention and nonintervention groups contain the exact same patients with exactly the same number and types of admissions with the only difference being the application of an attenuation factor in the simulated treated group. It is as if we have built a study not only with clonal genetic pairs of the people in each group, but as though we have somehow forced the clonal identicals to have identical experience in admissions and admission types so we could test the efficacy of the intervention. In the language of epidemiology, we are positing the perfect counterfactual, where the only difference between the two comparison groups is the intervention itself.

In the real world, observable savings evaluations compare groups with different proportions of people with different presenting diagnoses. We will now simulate this reality by creating groups of treated and controls without clonally identical diagnostic pairing. It is this heterogeneous group membership that is the substrate available for comparison in our real-world studies and we name the observable savings simulation. This simulation more realistically represents the variability to be expected in a real-world experiment or real-world budgetary observations by those responsible for committing organizational resources.

Observable Savings Simulation

- Demonstrate the expected observable impact of the intervention by creating two independent randomly selected populations of size (N=250).
- One group represents the treated with the random attenuator applied 50% of the time to those admissions deemed preventable.
- One group represents the untreated without any attenuation of cost.
- As in a real-world randomized clinical trial, the two groups will not have the same people the same number of times. Therefore, the preventable admission cases will be different in the treated and control groups.
- Calculate the savings between the control and the treated group.
- Repeat this 5,000 times.
- Sort order by the difference in savings.
- Calculate the savings percentiles.

For the 250-sample size, we now see at the mean 2.5th percentile not a savings but a cost of $4,968 per person enrolled. Increasing the sample size to 1,394 shows a mean 2.5th percentile per-person savings of $156. The average median savings for the two-sample size is $3,904 and $3,921, respectively. Compare these two numbers with the true average savings of the preventable admissions $(10,949,878/1,394)*0.5=3,928$. The observed best estimate (mean of medians) comes very close to the absolute true average value. This demonstrates that even with the additional noise of the heterogeneous comparison groups, the central tendency of the observable cost savings comes close to the truth.

Enrolling 250 patients would at the minimum observe a loss of $1,242,000 and at the median observe a savings of $976,000.

Enrolling 1,394 patients would at the minimum observe a savings of $217,464 and at the median observe a savings of $5,465,874.

The observed estimates demonstrate greater variability than the true savings because of the different patients and their differing admission histories in the treated and control groups. The median savings are pretty close to the true savings, but a CEO lives on the single instance he experiences, not the median of the 500,000 trials, so he must worry about the implications of the singleton experience for job tenure.

Keep in mind that we are only describing the cost savings of hospitalization without considering the additional costs of the interventions themselves.

The academic community, in planning a clinical trial, have a similar, although some might say a lower-stakes, version of this problem. A clinical trial is only permitted by the IRB if there is a reasonable chance (by convention 80%) that a statistically significant difference for a clinically meaningful observation could be detected. By convention this translates into an 80% chance of finding a difference that could not have occurred by chance 95% of the time.

This phrase could be translated in our simulation to be cost savings inclusive of intervention costs greater than zero at the 20th percentile. To increase power, you can increase the effectiveness of the intervention, increase the size of both the treated and control group, or increase the number of controls while keeping the treated number constant. For our clinical CEO, increasing intervention effectiveness means additional intervention resources.

Table 61 produces the percentile savings for a random seed of 169 and sample size of 250 in the treated, with a control size given by the ratio treated:control.

Table 61. Simulated observed cost savings per person (with different treated-to-control ratios †)

Ratio	Percentile 2.5%	10%	20%	21%	22%	50%	75%	90%
1:1	-5,194	-2,153	-199	-12	136	3,575	6,775	9,620
1:3	-3,426	-921	669	774	872	3,676	5,995	8,309
1:4	-3,407	-1,062	774	915	1,035	3,835	6,139	8,299

†Assumes 50% effectiveness of intervention on the preventable admissions (seed 169, N=250 treated, 5,000 trials).

In the 1:1 size ratio, at the 20th percentile, there is a net cost of $199 per person. The first instance of a cost savings is at the 22nd percentile ($136). By the 20th percentile power criteria, this study would be deemed inadequately powered. Power could be increased by increasing the size of the control group by extending the search for non-treated controls back in time to achieve a ratio of 1:3 (treated:control). Using this strategy, positive savings is achieved at the 20th percentile (+$669), thus achieving the desired power of 80%. Increasing the ratio of treated:control to 1:4 minimally improves power.

One could also improve power by increasing the number of treated with an equal number of controls (Table 62).

Table 62. Simulated savings per person; average of 100 seed simulations with 5,000 cost comparisons each †

	Observed	Cost	Savings	True Cost	Savings
Number per Group**	2.5th percentile	20th percentile	Median	Median	2.5th percentile
250	-4,968	95	3,904	3,865	2,522
697	-1,396	1,630	3,915	3,900	3,043
1,394	156	2,298	3,921	3,909	3,289
2,788	1,261	2,774	3,918	3,913	3,467

† 50% effectiveness of intervention for preventable admissions with equal-sized treated and control groups

The amount saved at the average 20th percentile increases. However, the total number of currently dialyzed patients is fixed, so in our case, the maximum matched treated:control group size is 697. To further increase the number of treated requires collaboration with another health care system, but in addition to the complexities of coordination and standardization between systems, this strategy dilutes the compelling nature of local data to drive local decisions.

Another solution to the power problem is to increase the follow-up observation time from one year to multiple years as power is driven by the number of admissions. Unfortunately, a longtime horizon is not an option for annual budgetary decisions.

Discussion

The power simulation of observable cost savings (Table 61) demonstrates that with a sample size of 250, even in the dialysis population example with a 20% modeled preventable admission waste and a 50% effective intervention, we could not expect an observed cost savings 21% of the time in a single year of follow-up. Requiring additional savings to cover intervention expenditures would push the break-even percentile upward before achieving a positive cost savings, further compromising power. It is not surprising, therefore, that in the natural course of events, CEOs will not spontaneously make any effort to achieve such unlikely observable savings.

The federal government or any payer with a large-enough patient population will benefit from true savings as they experience the average of all the program efforts. However, the federal government does not deliver care, and those who do, do not do it at scale with manifest savings to compel behavior.

Table 62 provides the information necessary to plan an intervention's budget. Built into its calculations is an explicit estimate of potential savings if all the identified preventable admissions are prevented. We then add a discount of 50% to compensate for overexuberance in identification of opportunity and delusional optimism of our implementation competence. We then must decide which of the columns is the most relevant one for budgetary planning.

Clearly, the true savings are known only to G-d as pure counterfactual and will not be visible in either a clinical trial or year-to-year budgetary comparisons. We need to look at the observed savings and probably use the convention that we could reasonably expect to achieve the observed 20th percentile. 80% of the time, we will save more per person than this amount. Our choice is akin to the academics' use of an 80% power decision point to justify proceeding with a study. Enroll 697 patients, and you will save $1,630 per person or $1,136,110 overall. Enroll 1,394 patients, and you will save $2,298 per person or $3,203,412 overall.

Now we have to decide whether we will design a comparison clinical trial study or just apply the intervention to everyone. Clearly, the savings are increased with the greater number of people enrolled, but this decision is somewhat subjective and context dependent, determined by the degree of certainty of effectiveness to justify proceeding without a clinical trial. Tightening up of sloppy administrative or care delivery practices falls into the category of not needing to do a trial. We do not demand a clinical trial to prove parachute efficacy before we refuse to jump out of a plane without one.[113] We do need clinical trials when we are blinded by the shiny object of technology without consideration of the health care system's response to that technology's signal.[114]

How could an inspired visionary CEO beat the risk and serve the public good? The solution is one introduced by John Bogle[115] many years ago: mutual funds with low overhead costs (the S&P 500 passive investment strategy). Spread your risk and costs across multiple initiatives, building common infrastructure for signal acquisition (patient call-in center), data analysis, and outreach using transferable institutional learning to keep costs low. Then assess a basket of intervention targets to increase the power to detect the average benefit overall. Someone on an institutional level must have the power and must sweat the details.

These details will include building self-service information creation resources[3,4,7,116] to identify, support, and promote the best of the institution's staff to evaluate, propose, intervene, and evaluate interventions. Develop interventions that first identify specific patient needs that have not been addressed for which you build a need-specific service offering. Partner with patients and educate them so that their neural nets (their brains) become the detector generating a signal to the learning health system for the preventable problem in evolution. Provide the patient with access to a responsive system of accountable health care traffic controllers able to initiate service delivery in real time and be held accountable for failures to act. Find those patients who slip through the surveillance web and interrogate them to determine why the system failed them and how it could be improved. Then instantiate those improvements.

Corporate dollars, consistent corporate will driving a vision of reusable shared resources and administrative care patterns, can bring the costs of any single intervention down and allow the activation and scaling of interventions so that by assessing the aggregation of these outcomes, local savings can be realized, recognized, and be institutionally reinforcing.

Population Health Inertia Induced by Misplaced NNT Individualism

The learning health system should make preventive interventions based on the best available evidence as well as clinical insight. How do the numbers needed to treat (NNT[73]) and individual benefit play out in the decision calculus?

An article by Wilson et al.[117] opines on the importance of the NNT in deciding whether to implement interventions. Let us use this article and its approach to explore. NNT is the number of patients needed to treat to prevent one bad outcome in the population presented in the reviewed medical study. The patient can then decide whether it is worth it to him to take the treatment. The NNT's purpose is to translate something complex into something understandable to doctors and patients alike. However, like all summaries, it is incomplete and, in some ways, corrupt. Consider the specific example cited.

> The NNT is a particularly meaningful metric in situations where a substantial relative treatment effect exists, but occurrence of outcomes is low. For example, the Systolic Blood Pressure Intervention Trial[118] was stopped early due to a marked observed treatment effect with a 5.2% occurrence of the composite cardiovascular end point in the intensive BP control group compared with 6.8% in the control group (P<.001). Although the relative effect size $[1-(5.2/6.8)=24\%]$ was large, the absolute effect size $(6.8-5.2)=1.6\%)$ led to an NNT of around 60, because the vast majority of patients do not experience any of the cardiovascular events in the composite outcome.[117]

The author focuses on the individual's benefit and individual's decision-making process, believing that since only a small number of patients will personally benefit, the majority of those patients will not want the intervention. Because the individual is inclined to reject the intervention, spending limited outreach dollars to achieve the small personal benefit is not a good use of limited funds, even if, at the population level, we could reduce the undesired outcome by 24%.

There are a couple of interesting issues unaddressed.

First, is it true that people will not expend resources for an unlikely personal outcome? We have a clear counterexample in the purchase of term life insurance by parents of young children. The parents know that they will survive beyond the term of the insurance, and the insurance companies are betting on that, as well. So term life is, from an investment perspective, a loser's bet. Or is it? What is the goal? Protection. What are you protecting against? The loss of financial support for a family when their breadwinner has died is so awful that the good that is achieved in protecting against this awful but extremely rare event is worth the cost. No insurance salesman stresses the rarity of the event or the badness of the investment because it is not an investment. No return is expected. The salesman stresses the awfulness of the event. The preventive medicine intervention follows a similar logic. In fact, the observed reduction of 24% of the cardiovascular endpoint was deemed so clinically important and clearly statistically significant that the trial was stopped prematurely.

Second, the NNT summary hides a truth stated explicitly in the quoted paragraph.

I will give you a moment to review that paragraph again to find the other truth hidden in plain sight.

The study was stopped early. More effect would have been seen if even the original design had been respected and the study continued. However, it was not ethical on an individual level to proceed with the placebo arm because both clinical and statistical significance had been achieved. The goal of the study could not get beyond this effectiveness barrier. Once an NNT of 1 in 60 was achieved, no further study was permissible, so the 1 in 60 is an underestimate of the effectiveness even as designed.

Now we assume that the positive finding has a biologic correlate. We have changed something biologically that was causal of the clinical observation. That imputed cause is available for us to consider in our intervention planning. We might model reality that once this cause is in place, we would expect continued improvement with prolongation of the intervention. We might model the reality as a continuum where greater control, either longer in duration or greater in magnitude, as in the reduction of blood pressure, might result in a better outcome. Neither is proven by the study, but it is up to us to decide how to draw broad inference for public intervention or whether to be concretely bound to the early terminated result.

The article goes on to describe how it would be better to have more personalized information that could make the promised return higher than 1/60 at the individual level. The truth is that any decision rule—like any laboratory test—would have a sensitivity, specificity, and a positive and negative predictive value. Those responsible for population health care implementation strategy must consider how many people they are willing to treat to capture the percent of the population who would benefit. There will always be a tradeoff.

In addition, there are subpopulations whose outcomes are grossly deviant from the general population in baseline risk. We see racial and economic disparities in outcomes and wonder whether the cause for these disparities goes beyond the usual risk factors entered as lone freestanding risk factors but rather somehow are catalyzed by social, environmental, or biologic factors. This functional interaction effect on the risk factors might require a more aggressive intervention approach than commonly used.

This logic applied in the management of LDL cholesterol in our medical group is illustrative. Suppose having recognized that the Bronx has the worst cardiovascular and stroke mortality of all 60 counties in New York State, we proposed that all adults 40–75 years of age in our clinics be treated with lipid-lowering agents to achieve targets of <70? There is no randomized literature supporting this approach in primary prevention. But suppose we decided that the present reality of stroke and cardiovascular disease in the Bronx is unacceptable, and we make the decision to bring the population to an LDL level that is much lower than national standards. How many people would be included?

1. Primary care MMG age 40–75 in 2018 with an LDL value within two years of outpatient visit: N=84,842
2. With LDL within 2 years of outpatient visit of greater than 70: N= 78,109
3. With LDL within 2 years of outpatient visit greater than 100: N= 58,188

The decision cannot be made lightly, and clearly the myositis risk, although low, will need to be shared with the population. What is the institutional machinery that needs to be invoked—institutional ethics, convening local experts? What agreement must be sought from the practicing physicians? When you have the ability to see the consequences of health system practice and patient choices, you have an obligation to intervene and make best judgement decisions. The procedure that should be followed is unexplored territory.

Ethical Implications: Noblesse Oblige or Well-Defended Neglect

A learning health system, by virtue of its potential to ask, answer, plan, and implement, has an ethical portfolio that is distinct from its clinical participants. Sins of both omission and commission are possible at a scale unimagined in the classic patient-to-single-practitioner ethics space. There are ways to defend against the potential for infinite ethical demand and cost, none of which are admirable. We will innumerate some here.

One can choose not to look. Choosing to not look can be accomplished in many ways—some are subtler than others.

1. Not to fund the creation of a data repository.
2. Not to fund the availability of real tools that can easily build cohorts and outcomes[7] but to hide behind the appearance of capability with standard inadequate slicing-and-dicing EMR tools that do not creating meaningful accountabilities only possible with identified temporally enriched cohorts and outcomes.[3]
3. Not to require the use of the tools by staff in different departments as part of operational professional competence to find problems and evaluate remediation efforts.

After an institution has built the capability to look and has created the operational impetus for its departments to spontaneously and creatively ask questions, it then has to decide when to act using scarce resources.

Here we have a number of clever defenses supportive of inertia. Inertia is a benefit budgetarily as it does not require expenditures of scarce nonreimbursable dollars. There is a perverse incentive to develop clever defenses against this unfortunate, noisome budgetary demand.

Defense number one is that we do not know enough, and until we know more, we should not change our practice. We must wait. By a careful, concrete fealty only to "the proven," as described in the previous chapter, the LHS can obviate expenditure of time and effort. In that chapter I argued for a more expansive view of the considerations. I suspect, however, even if you restrict yourself to the provable, there is a lot to be done.

Defense number two is to invoke ethics as a barrier. In any population health decision, there are both risks and benefits. Since resources are scarce, someone must make priority decisions balancing risks and benefits. Today, the word "paternalism" has a bad odor, and to obviate this charge, does the learning health system have to wait for the request to come from the patient population? Is it sufficient for the LHS to make a best judgement and inform the population through a webpage of the policy and protocol, permitting those who wish to opt out upon their request but not requiring a discussion with every patient? The energy that would be spent on a prolonged discussion with frankly only the appearance of engagement might be better spent in assuring adherence to medication. Polling the patients to determine their preferences is an insuperable barrier to action.

The whole purpose of representative democracy is premised on the notion that the populace is too busy to invest the time and energy to learn and to construct legislation. The people need to elect representatives to do this for them and have the opportunity to remove such representatives when they do not serve their purposes. The LHS is similar to a city manager. While not elected, the LHS is hired by the people it serves to make decisions while still providing transparency for its decisions and provide meaningful opportunities to learn about the intrinsic benefits and risks.

Note that this may not be informed consent, as the individual is given the opportunity to avail himself of the information, but there is no responsibility for the LHS to demonstrate that the patient was made aware of risk and benefits and consented to specific intervention. The patient, if he goes to the website and avails himself himself of the opportunity to learn of risks and benefits, will, in that same opportunity, learn of the opportunity to opt out should he wish to do so. Most people will not avail themselves of the opportunity and as a result will functionally be opted in by default.

To some, this plan will seem odd. A premium has historically been placed on personal communication of risks and benefits to the patient, with the patient being the autonomous agent once educated. For benefits that come with a high risk, there is a clear imperative for this one-on-one decision making. But there are many decisions made for the patient in practice that do not require endless conversation.

Consider tradeoffs made in the sensitivity and specificity of automated laboratory tests. Consider tradeoffs made in sterilization solutions and their dwell time. There are many decisions that are paternalistically—or, rather, properly—deferred to others so as not to overwhelm the individual patient or encumber the delivery system with unlimited conversations. The ethics of the LHS include deciding which of these decisions need to be a part of the short patient encounter and at what cost—the cost being more than the time expended but also the functional success or lack thereof of implementing the proper intervention on the largest number of people. Admittedly, there is subjectivity here, and as a society, we have not engaged this question fully, but this ethical consideration is an inevitable feature of a learning health system.

The LHS, by its very nature, has a duty of the old noblesse oblige. Its role is to establish policies for the outreach and delivery of care using the best available information from randomized controlled trials (RCTs) and best practices determined by meaningful review and extrapolation by reasonably trained experts. Its decisions should not be constrained by the RCT data limits. It must be permitted—nay, required—to use best judgment publicly stated using model-based extrapolation as long as the decision is documented with its supporting thoughts available for public review at any time.

Worked Example: Who Should Be Treated with High-Dose Statin in the Medical Group in 2018?

Given the state of incomplete knowledge and the ethical imperative to intervene on a public health issue, let us work through an example using data from 2018 MMG medical group and enter into a Socratic dialogue with our colleagues on how we should proceed.

The first colleague states with absolute certainty that since we know that high-intensity lipid therapy can arrest the biologic progression of atherosclerotic cardiovascular disease (ASCVD) and can prevent in higher-risk patients from a new onset of myocardial infarction,[119-121] it makes sense to treat everybody in our population of patients—inner-city minority patients—with high-dose statin and to do so to target LDL levels less than 70.

This position argues that even if the literature does not yet justify treatment to target, in its pathetic focus on the 10-year risk, we have enough experience of the effectiveness of the clinically ill and enough understanding of the natural history with its cumulative aggregation of lipid endothelial damage to justify broad efforts to reduce LDL even in patients who will not have immediate clinically obvious sequelae in the next 10 years but who clearly are collecting fatty streaks in their endothelium and developing the damage that will inevitably lead over decades to coronary events. This natural history has been known since the 1950s when lipid streaks were visible in the postmortem arteries of young men killed in the Korean War.

Why should we aggressively target LDLs of 70, and why should we broadly apply this intervention? Two reasons. First, lower must be better, and whatever concern one might have about side effects can be cause for early cessation but not cause for failure to initiate therapy. The side effects are relatively mild and easy to detect prior to serious consequences, and when stopped, the adverse event usually subsides. Second, as a practical matter, uniform policies of application have a better chance of implementation and maintenance than targeted efforts. Experience in universal precautions in infectious disease with universal contact precautions with blood is such an example. Whenever you try to tailor interventions to subpopulations, there are implementation challenges. The justification of such tailoring is cost or side effects that are intolerable or side effects that, once manifest, cannot be eliminated.

This approach is countered by another physician who says that we can only do what is proven to be clinically effective in clinical population studies. Even if I concede that the side effects are manageable and that we can stop the medication before irreversible consequences occur, I will not undertake any intervention that is not fully substantiated by explicit clinical trial in populations like mine.[122] Moreover, I do not accept the treatment to target LDL as we have no proof of this yet. I have made the argument purposely sharp and focused on the proven randomized control trial, allowing no room for judgment to drive a population health decision.

Now this position, although some might think has been presented as a straw man, actually can be articulated with a degree of intellectual rigor.[123] Hayward claims that the randomized control trials have functionally only been randomized to high- and low-dose statins, not to specific targeted values of LDL. As a result, attempts to draw inferences from the achieved LDL levels in those studies with the certainty accorded to RCT evidence is incorrect. The LDL level achieved is not the result of a randomized study goal but rather an artifact of an observation. Its quality of evidence is reduced to that of an observational study, not to its parent RCT in which it is embedded. As an observational study, alternative confounding explanations must be explicitly identified and eliminated before invoking the "lower is better" hypothesis.

An alternative hypothesis is the pleiotropic effects of the statins on inflammation, thrombosis, and oxidation as plausible mechanism for mediating the benefits of statin therapy, not the LDL-lowering effect. He goes further to suggest that in this observational sub-study, the LDL lowering is actually a marker for compliance, so we are merely observing that those with greater compliance do better than those with less. Compliance, by the way, not only achieves the alternative hypothesis direct pleiotropic effect but also selects for the compliant population. It is well known in placebo trials that those who are compliant with a placebo do better than those who are not placebo compliant.

One realizes that given these two strong positions, it seems to some to be prudent to punt the decision to an in-depth, informed conversation between patient and physician. Consider for a moment how much time the physician has, how complicated the issues being considered are, and how this decision to punt is functionally a decision for inertia. Of course, sometimes inertia is not a bad thing. As we have learned in medical school, *primum no nocere*, but if you are of the first opinion, the inertia posing as patient autonomy is both wrong and unethical.

We will not resolve this controversy here, but let's for a moment evaluate our care in light of the assumed truth that lower is better and that a target goal of <70 is critical. Using this criterion and looking at diabetics cared for in 2018 in our medical group, how well are we doing? By reviewing our care in this unforgiving light, we will make clear why a central ethical decision might have legs.

Let us use as a fact base information available from Sean P. Kane ClinCalc,[124] a website that provides useful clinical tools to calculate risk as well as summaries of medication recommendations. Similar work can be found in commercial work of UpToDate.

For the purpose of this dialogue, we are going to assume the following people should be treated with intensive lipid lowering therapy.

- Individuals with clinical ASCVD
- Individuals with primary elevations of LDL≥190 mg/dL
- Individuals 40–75 years of age with diabetes and an LDL 70–189 mg/dL without clinical ASCVD
- Individuals without clinical ASCVD or diabetes who are 40–75 years of age with LDL 70–189 mg/dL and a 10-year ASCVD risk of 7.5% or higher

We are going to assume as fact that for the groups identified above, the high-intensity regimen is required (atorvastatin 80 mg) and that we should be treating to target LDL<70, so if the target laboratory value goal is not achieved, prescriptions of doses below the maximum of the high-intensity statin regimen are to be considered inadequate therapy.

This is a quick and dirty calculation and does not allow for individualization, but we are approaching the clinical care learning health system policy from a public health perspective and want to simulate the implications of this approach.

MMG general information with focus on diabetics

The following data will be used to assess the adequacy of our efforts at lipid control in patients with incontrovertible need of therapy.

- Primary care MMG age 40–75 in 2018   N=95,800
  - With LDL within 24 hours of outpatient visit greater than 100   N=28,872
  - With LDL within 24 hours of outpatient visit of greater than 70   N=42,192
    - With LDL>70 and HgbA1c≥6.5 in the preceding 5 years   N=12,484
      - Diabetics with no statin (Figure 71)   N=4,538
      - Diabetics with inadequate statins (*Table 63*)   N=7,180

In 2018, according to approach #1, of 12,484 diabetics age 40–75 in the medical group, 11,718 (93%) were inadequately treated. Of course, we cannot account for legitimate decisions not to increase doses or patient noncompliance, but as a clinical service in the worst county in New York State for stroke and cardiovascular disease, a clinical population-based approach would be appropriate.

These patients all fit into the current guidelines for therapy or for intensification, and we should note that of the 42,192 patients who currently have an LDL recorded, 11,718 (28%) are diabetics with inadequate statin coverage. Universal institution of treatment with intensification of all diabetics in the MMG clinic with an LDL >70 would immediately yield an additional 11,718 of 12,484, constituting 93% of our diabetically eligible patients.

To achieve this huge target apparently requires more than individual counseling. While we have never claimed to be a perfect LHS, we can reasonably assert, given our decades of commitment to assuming managed care risk in this population, that we are at least at the median of care-quality performance nationally. Thus, this issue surfaced in this chapter is of much broader concern than just to the population of the Bronx.

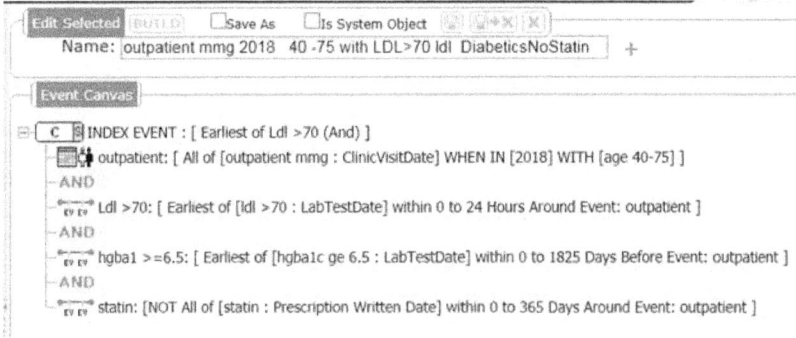

Figure 71. MMG diabetics LDL>70 on no statins (2018)

Now apply the statin approach to the entire medical group to understand the implications of our assumptions.

Executive Summary (for Those Who Cannot Wait)

- 48% of patients aged 40–75 in MMG in 2018 are candidates for intensive lipid-lowering therapy
- 79.5% of these patients do not achieve target LDL<70
- Of those who do not achieve the target, 91.5% are at submaximal doses of statin therapy.

Actual Workup

1. In 2018, the MMG group had 95,800 people between the ages of 40 and 75.
2. 84,851 had a lipid-level determination within two years of the clinic visit.
   a. 16,514 (19.4%) had evidence by diagnosis of atherosclerotic cardiovascular disease in the antecedent 10 years (Appendix C).
   b. 5,385 (6.1%) had evidence of LDL≥190 in the 10 years before the first clinic visit in 2018.

Table 63. Submaximal statin therapy in MMG diabetics with LDL>70 (2018)

Medication and Dose	Count	Not Maximal Therapy
ATORVASTATIN 40 MG TABLET	1807	1807
ATORVASTATIN 20 MG TABLET	1563	1563
ATORVASTATIN 10 MG TABLET	990	990
ATORVASTATIN 80 MG TABLET	825	
SIMVASTATIN 20 MG TABLET	650	650
SIMVASTATIN 40 MG TABLET	569	569
PRAVASTATIN 40 MG TABLET	251	251
SIMVASTATIN 10 MG TABLET	225	225
PRAVASTATIN 20 MG TABLET	203	203
ROSUVASTATIN 20 MG TABLET	184	184
ROSUVASTATIN 10 MG TABLET	169	169
ROSUVASTATIN 40 MG TABLET	126	126
ROSUVASTATIN 5 MG TABLET	99	99
PRAVASTATIN 80 MG TABLET	70	70
PRAVASTATIN 10 MG TABLET	62	62
LOVASTATIN 40 MG TABLET	62	62
LOVASTATIN 20 MG TABLET	60	60
SIMVASTATIN 5 MG TABLET	24	24
SIMVASTATIN 80 MG TABLET	18	18
LOVASTATIN 10 MG TABLET	14	14
PITAVASTATIN CALCIUM 2 MG TABLET	6	6
CRESTOR 20 MG TABLET	4	4
AMLODIPINE 5 MG-ATORVASTATIN 40 MG TABLET	3	3
PITAVASTATIN CALCIUM 4 MG TABLET	3	3
AMLODIPINE 10 MG-ATORVASTATIN 80 MG TABLET	2	2
PITAVASTATIN CALCIUM 1 MG TABLET	2	2
CRESTOR 40 MG TABLET	2	
LIPITOR 80 MG TABLET	2	
FLUVASTATIN ER 80 MG TABLET,EXTENDED RELEASE 24 HR	2	2
CRESTOR 5 MG TABLET	1	1
LOVASTATIN ER 20 MG TABLET,EXTENDED RELEASE 24 HR	1	1
CRESTOR 10 MG TABLET	1	1
EZETIMIBE 10 MG-ATORVASTATIN 20 MG TABLET	1	1
AMLODIPINE 10 MG-ATORVASTATIN 10 MG TABLET	1	1
AMLODIPINE 5 MG-ATORVASTATIN 10 MG TABLET	1	1
AMLODIPINE 5 MG-ATORVASTATIN 20 MG TABLET	1	1
LIPITOR 10 MG TABLET	1	1
FLUVASTATIN 20 MG CAPSULE	1	1
PRAVACHOL 40 MG TABLET	1	1
ZOCOR 40 MG TABLET	1	1
AMLODIPINE 5 MG-ATORVASTATIN 80 MG TABLET	1	1
AMLODIPINE 10 MG-ATORVASTATIN 40 MG TABLET	1	1
(blank)		
Grand Total	8009	7180

    c. 16,309 diabetic patients using the case definition of HgbA1c≥6.5 without a diagnosis of atherosclerotic vascular disease in the previous 10 years, nor LDL≥190, but with one of the following three indicia of complicating condition (see method in Appendix A).

      i.   Hypertension by virtue of either a systolic blood pressure greater than or equal to 140 or hypertension medication prescribed

      ii.   Chronic kidney disease GFR<60

      iii.   BMI≥30 (my proxy for metabolic syndrome)

   d.   951 additional patients with diabetes (1% of the entire population of patients) but who did not have evidence in the EMR of the three complicating conditions, atherosclerotic cardiovascular disease, or LDL≥190.

Groups A, B, and C are assumed to require aggressive lipid lowering with either achieving an LDL<70 or using maximal statin therapy atorvastatin 80mg or rosuvastatin 40mg daily.

The pooled cohort equation for cardiovascular risk[125] was applied to those patients not in Groups A, B, or C. (Please note: the error in the equation in the primary article is corrected in the supplement.) This yielded the following:

- 2,713 people with a 10-year cardiovascular risk of >20%
- 15,044 with a 10-year cardiovascular risk of >7.5%

An argument could be made for intensive therapy even for those with a 10-year risk of >7.5%, but for the purpose of this exercise, I will choose the >20% so there can be no concern about exaggeration of the problem.

Restricting to those in Groups A, B, and C and the additional 2,713 with a calculated risk of 20% in the next 10 years, I have therefore identified 40,921 patients who require intensive therapy and will evaluate the quality of the care we are providing against the standard described.

Keep in mind, this conservative approach identifies 40,921 of the 84,851 40–75-year-olds in the medical group as needing intensive therapy. This is 48% of the entire cohort.

Now let's review how well we are doing.

Looking at the last available LDL, we find that only 8,407 have achieve an LDL<70 (Table 64).

From an LDL perspective, there are 32,512 of the 40,921 or 79.5% who do not achieve the target LDL.

The actual statin medication and dose used for the patients we have identified who need intensive therapy but are not at LDL goal is provided in Table 65.

Table 64. LDL findings

LDL test range	Frequency	Percent
0–70	8,407	21
70–100	12,085	30
≥100	20,037	49
Not available	390	1

Table 65. Statin dose for patients needing intensive therapy

Product	Freq	Per cent
	11541	35.5
atorvastatin 40 mg tablet	4765	14.66
atorvastatin 20 mg tablet	3757	11.56
atorvastatin 80 mg tablet	2483	7.64
atorvastatin 10 mg tablet	2252	6.93
simvastatin 20 mg tablet	1553	4.78
simvastatin 40 mg tablet	1417	4.36
pravastatin 40 mg tablet	662	2.04
pravastatin 20 mg tablet	585	1.8
simvastatin 10 mg tablet	568	1.75
rosuvastatin 20 mg tablet	567	1.74
rosuvastatin 10 mg tablet	546	1.68
NA	390	1.2
rosuvastatin 40 mg tablet	310	0.95
rosuvastatin 5 mg tablet	300	0.92
pravastatin 80 mg tablet	184	0.57
pravastatin 10 mg tablet	168	0.52
lovastatin 40 mg tablet	164	0.5
lovastatin 20 mg tablet	128	0.39
simvastatin 80 mg tablet	57	0.18
simvastatin 5 mg tablet	50	0.15
lovastatin 10 mg tablet	29	0.09
pitavastatin calcium 2 mg tablet	12	0.04
pitavastatin calcium 4 mg tablet	8	0.02
pitavastatin calcium 1 mg tablet	5	0.02
fluvastatin 40 mg capsule	4	0.01
fluvastatin ER 80 mg tablet, extended release 24 hr	3	0.01
fluvastatin 20 mg capsule	2	0.01
lovastatin ER 20 mg tablet, extended release 24 hr	1	0
lovastatin ER 40 mg tablet, extended release 24 hr	1	0

Reviewing the last statin prescription written to see how many of them are at maximal dose (either atorvastatin 80 or rosuvastatin 40), we find only 2,793 of the 32,512 or only 8.5% are on maximal doses.

Appendix A. CLG Identification of Patients Either with LDL≥190 or Diabetics with One of Three Complicating Diagnoses. No Patient with Dx of Atherosclerotic Vascular Disease.

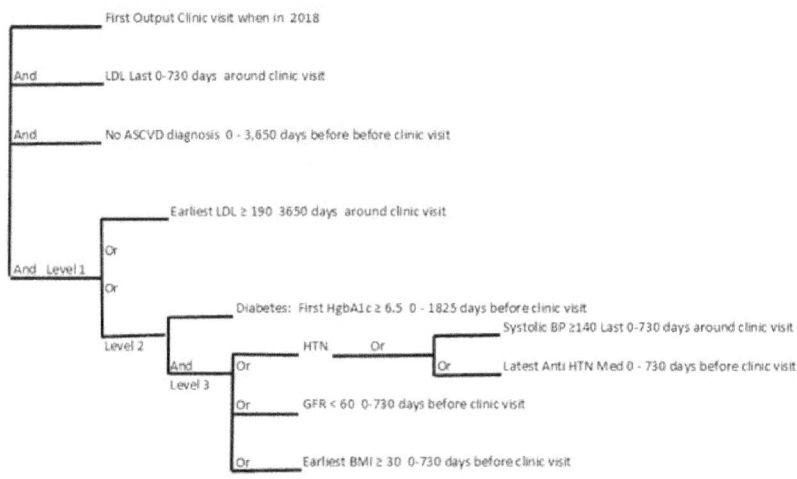

Edit Selected | Build | Save As | Is System Object | | + X | X

Name: mmg1840-75LdlgroupedNoAscvdLevelone[2 I3

Event Canvas

- ⊟ C INDEX EVENT : [Latest of LDL (And)]
  - mmg 40-75: [Earliest of [outpt MMG : ClinicVisitDate] WHEN IN [2018] WITH [age 40-75]]
  - AND
  - LDL: [Latest of [LDL : LabTestDate] within 0 to 730 Days Around Event: mmg 40-75]
  - AND
  - ascvd: [NOT All of [diagnosis ascvd : ICDDiagnosisAdmitDate] within 0 to 3650 Days Before Event: mmg 40-75]
  - AND
  - ⊟ (. . .) level One: [Earliest of Any (Or)]
    - LDL> =190: [Earliest of [LDL ge 190 : LabTestDate] within 0 to 3650 Days Around Event: mmg 40-75]
    - OR
    - ⊟ (. . .) Level 2: [Earliest of Any (And)]
      - hgba1c ge 6.5: [Earliest of [hgbA1c ge 6.5 : LabTestDate] within 0 to 1825 Days Before Event: mmg 40-75]
      - AND
      - ⊟ (. . .) level 3: [Earliest of Any (Or)]
        - ⊟ (. . .) Htn: [Earliest of Any (Or)]
          - BPsys ge 140: [Earliest of [bp svs ge 140 : FindingDate] within 0 to 730 Days Before Event: mmg 40-75]
          - OR
          - antiHtnMed: [All of [prescription written antiHtn : Prescription Written Date] within 0 to 730 Days Before Event: mmg 40-75]
        - OR
        - Gfr <60: [Earliest of [gfr <60 : LabTestDate] within 0 to 730 Days Before Event: mmg 40-75]
        - OR
        - BMI ge 30: [Earliest of [BMI ge 30 : FindingDate] within 0 to 730 Days Before Event: mmg 40-75]

Simplified Structure

Cohort: Index eventline points to : First Output Clinic Visit

First Output Clinic visit when in 2018

And LDL Last 0-730 days around clinic visit

And No ASCVD diagnosis 0 - 3,650 days before before clinic visit

Earliest LDL ≥ 190 3650 days around clinic visit

And Level 1 Or Or

Level 2

Diabetes: First HgbA1c ≥ 6.5 0 - 1825 days before clinic visit

Systolic BP ≥140 Last 0-730 days around clinic visit

And Level 3 Or HTN Or Or Latest Anti HTN Med 0 - 730 days before clinic visit

Or GFR < 60 0-730 days before clinic visit

Or Earliest BMI ≥ 30 0-730 days before clinic visit

Appendix B. No ASCVD, No LDL≥190, Diabetics Without a Complicating HTN, Renal Insufficiency, or Obesity

Edit Selected ⬚⬚⬚⬚ ☐Save As ☐Is System Object ⬚ ⬚ ⇒X: X
Name: mmg1840-75LdlgroupedNoAscvdLevelonel2 l3noLdlge190nos3

Event Canvas

C B INDEX EVENT : [Earliest of mmg 40-75 (And)]
- mmg 40-75: [Earliest of [outpt MMG : ClinicVisitDate] WHEN IN [2018] WITH [age 40-75]]
- AND
- LDL: [Latest of [LDL : LabTestDate] within 0 to 730 Days Around Event: mmg 40-75]
- AND
- ascvd: [NOT All of [diagnosis ascvd : ICDDiagnosisAdmitDate] within 0 to 3650 Days Before Event: mmg 40-75]
- AND
- (...) level One: [Earliest of Any (Or)]
  - (...) Level 2: [Earliest of Any (And)]
    - hgba1c ge 6.5: [Earliest of [hgbA1c ge 6.5 : LabTestDate] within 0 to 1825 Days Before Event: mmg 40-75]
    - AND
    - (...) level 3: [NOT All of Any (Or)]
      - (...) Htn: [Earliest of Any (Or)]
        - BPsys ge 140: [Earliest of [bp sys ge 140 : FindingDate] within 0 to 730 Days Before Event: mmg 40-75]
        - OR
        - antiHtnMed: [All of [prescription written antiHtn : Prescription Written Date] within 0 to 730 Days Before Event: mmg 40-75]
      - OR
      - Gfr <60: [Earliest of [gfr <60 : LabTestDate] within 0 to 730 Days Before Event: mmg 40-75]
      - OR
      - BMI ge 30: [Earliest of [BMI ge 30 : FindingDate] within 0 to 730 Days Before Event: mmg 40-75]
- AND
- LDL>=190: [NOT All of [LDL ge 190 : LabTestDate] within 0 to 3650 Days Around Event: mmg 40-75]

Appendix C. Diagnoses Indicative of Atherosclerotic Cardiovascular Disease

Row Labels	Count of ICD Diagnosis
414.01-CORONARY ATHEROSCLEROSIS,NATIVE CORONARY VESSEL	2781
I25.10-Atherosclerotic heart disease of native coronary artery without angina pectoris	1871
443.9-PERIPH VASCULAR DIS NOS	1461
414-OTH CHR ISCHEMIC HRT DIS	1167
434.91-CEREBRAL ART OCCL, UNSPEC, W/CEREB INFARCT	889
I73.9-Peripheral vascular disease, unspecified	792
414.00-CORONARY ATHEROSCLEROSIS;UNSPEC TYPE,NATIVE/GRAFT	770
411.1-INTERMED CORONARY SYND	664
412-OLD MYOCARDIAL INFARCT	548
440.21-ATHEROSCLEROSIS,NATIVE ARTERIES,EXTREM W/INT CLAUD	493
440.0-AORTIC ATHEROSCLEROSIS	423
I63.9-Cerebral infarction, unspecified	306
436-CVA	303
410.71-SUBENDO INFRC-INIT EPISD	303
440-ATHEROSCLEROSIS	298
433.10-OCCL & STEN, CAROTID ART, W/O CEREB INFARCT	211
414.9-CHR ISCHEMIC HRT DIS NOS	183
440.22-ATHEROSCLEROSIS,NATIVE ARTERIES,EXTREM W/REST PAIN	171
I25.2-Old myocardial infarction	163
I21.4-Non-ST elevation (NSTEMI) myocardial infarction	135
I25.110-Atherosclerotic heart disease of native coronary artery with unstable angina pectoris	134
433.1-OCCLUSION & STENOSIS OF THE CAROTID ARTERY	123
I25.119-Atherosclerotic heart disease of native coronary artery with unspecified angina pectoris	117
I63.8-Other cerebral infarction	115
440.23-ATHEROSCLEROSIS,NATIVE ARTERIES,EXTREM W/ULCERAT.	92
414.8-CHR ISCHEMIC HRT DIS NEC	80
410.91-AMI NOS-INITIAL EPISODE	77
434.90-CEREBRAL ART OCCL, UNSPEC, W/O CEREB INFARCT	58
434.9-CEREBRAL ARTERY OCCLUSION, UNSPECIFIED	56
434.11-CEREBRAL EMBOLISM WITH CEREBRAL INFARCTION	56
I25.118-Atherosclerotic heart disease of native coronary artery with other forms of angina pectoris	54
I69.959-Hemiplegia and hemiparesis following unspecified cerebrovascular disease affecting unspecified side	52
410.11-ANTER AMI NEC-INIT EPISD	49
410.90-AMI NOS-EPISODE NOS	49
440.9-ATHEROSCLEROSIS NOS	48
I21.3-ST elevation (STEMI) myocardial infarction of unspecified site	47
I69.354-Hemiplegia and hemiparesis following cerebral infarction affecting left non-dominant side	46
Z95.1-Presence of aortocoronary bypass graft	44
410.41-INFER AMI NEC-INIT EPISD	43
410.9-MYOCARDIAL INFARCT NOS	42
440.4-CHRONIC TOTAL OCCLUSION OF ARTERY OF THE EXTREMITI	40
I21.19-ST elevation (STEMI) myocardial infarction involving other coronary artery of inferior wall	38
I69.351-Hemiplegia and hemiparesis following cerebral infarction affecting right dominant side	37
440.20-ATHEROSCLEROSIS,NATIVE ARTERIES OF EXTREM.,UNSPEC.	33
746.85-CORONARY ARTERY ANOMALY	33
433.11-OCCL & STEN, CAROTID ART, W/CEREB INFARCT	32
I25.5-Ischemic cardiomyopathy	31
440.1-RENAL ARTERY ATHEROSCLER	30

I25.83-Coronary atherosclerosis due to lipid rich plaque	4
I21.9-Acute myocardial infarction, unspecified	4
I63.10-Cerebral infarction due to embolism of unspecified precerebral artery	4
I63.20-Cerebral infarction due to unspecified occlusion or stenosis of unspecified precerebral arteries	4
433.80-OCCL & STEN, OTHER PRECEREB ART, W/O CEREB INFARCT	4
I63.432-Cerebral infarction due to embolism of left posterior cerebral artery	4
I69.151-Hemiplegia and hemiparesis following nontraumatic intracerebral hemorrhage affecting right dominant	4
I63.311-Cerebral infarction due to thrombosis of right middle cerebral artery	4
I63.212-Cerebral infarction due to unspecified occlusion or stenosis of left vertebral artery	4
I69.328-Other speech and language deficits following cerebral infarction	4
Z95.820-Peripheral vascular angioplasty status with implants and grafts	4
I63.531-Cerebral infarction due to unspecified occlusion or stenosis of right posterior cerebral artery	4
414.11-ANEURYSM OF CORONARY VESSELS	4
I63.02-Cerebral infarction due to thrombosis of basilar artery	4
I63.239-Cerebral infarction due to unspecified occlusion or stenosis of unspecified carotid artery	3
I69.393-Ataxia following cerebral infarction	3
410.40-INFER AMI NEC-EPISOD NOS	3
I63.419-Cerebral infarction due to embolism of unspecified middle cerebral artery	3
I63.22-Cerebral infarction due to unspecified occlusion or stenosis of basilar artery	3
I63.421-Cerebral infarction due to embolism of right anterior cerebral artery	3
Q27.9-Congenital malformation of peripheral vascular system, unspecified	3
434.10-CEREBRAL EMBOLISM W/O CEREBRAL INFARCTION	3
434-CEREBRAL ARTERY OCCLUS	3
410.7-SUBENDOCARDIAL INFARCT	3
I69.851-Hemiplegia and hemiparesis following other cerebrovascular disease affecting right dominant side	3
I63.89-Other cerebral infarction	3
I69.998-Other sequelae following unspecified cerebrovascular disease	3
433.30-OCCL & STEN, MULT & BILAT ART, W/O CEREB INFARCT	3
433.81-OCCL & STEN, OTHER PRECEREB ART, W/CEREB INFARCT	3
I69.154-Hemiplegia and hemiparesis following nontraumatic intracerebral hemorrhage affecting left non-domina	3
434.00-CEREBRAL THROMBOSIS W/O CEREBRAL INFARCTION	3
410.12-ANTER AMI NEC-LATR EPISD	3
414.04-CORONARY ATHEROSCLEROSIS OF ARTERY BYPASS GRAFT	3
414.4-Cor ath d/t calc cor lsn	3
I69.320-Aphasia following cerebral infarction	3
I63.39-Cerebral infarction due to thrombosis of other cerebral artery	2
I63.59-Cerebral infarction due to unspecified occlusion or stenosis of other cerebral artery	2
I63.541-Cerebral infarction due to unspecified occlusion or stenosis of right cerebellar artery	2
I69.198-Other sequelae of nontraumatic intracerebral hemorrhage	2
414.2-CHRONIC TOTAL OCCLUSION OF CORONARY ARTERY	2
I69.254-Hemiplegia and hemiparesis following other nontraumatic intracranial hemorrhage affecting left non-d	2
I22.2-Subsequent non-ST elevation (NSTEMI) myocardial infarction	2
I69.298-Other sequelae of other nontraumatic intracranial hemorrhage	2
I63.232-Cerebral infarction due to unspecified occlusion or stenosis of left carotid arteries	2
I25.709-Atherosclerosis of coronary artery bypass graft(s), unspecified, with unspecified angina pectoris	2
410.02-ANTEROLAT AMI-LATR EPISD	2
I69.319-Unspecified symptoms and signs involving cognitive functions following cerebral infarction	2
I63.449-Cerebral infarction due to embolism of unspecified cerebellar artery	2
414.05-CORONARY ATHEROSCLEROSIS OF UNSPEC.TYPE BYPASS GFT	2
I25.700-Atherosclerosis of coronary artery bypass graft(s), unspecified, with unstable angina pectoris	2
I51.5-Myocardial degeneration	2
I69.91-Cognitive deficits following unspecified cerebrovascular disease	2
433.2-OCCLUSION & STENOSIS OF THE VERTEBRAL ARTERY	2
410.51-LATRL AMI NEC-INIT EPISD	2

I69.352-Hemiplegia and hemiparesis following cerebral infarction affecting left dominant side   2
I69.993-Ataxia following unspecified cerebrovascular disease   2
I25.811-Atherosclerosis of native coronary artery of transplanted heart without angina pectoris   2
433.21-OCCL & STEN OF VERTEBRAL ART, W/CEREB INFARCT   2
I63.132-Cerebral infarction due to embolism of left carotid artery   2
I21.21-ST elevation (STEMI) myocardial infarction involving left circumflex coronary artery   2
I63.139-Cerebral infarction due to embolism of unspecified carotid artery   2
T82.856A-Stenosis of peripheral vascular stent, initial encounter   2
I63.522-Cerebral infarction due to unspecified occlusion or stenosis of left anterior cerebral artery   2
I63.342-Cerebral infarction due to thrombosis of left cerebellar artery   2
I21.A1-Myocardial infarction type 2   2
440.32-ATHEROSCLEROSIS;NONAUTOL BIO BYPASS GRAFT;EXTREM.   2
I63.422-Cerebral infarction due to embolism of left anterior cerebral artery   2
I69.193-Ataxia following nontraumatic intracerebral hemorrhage   2
I69.898-Other sequelae of other cerebrovascular disease   2
I25.89-Other forms of chronic ischemic heart disease   2
I69.854-Hemiplegia and hemiparesis following other cerebrovascular disease affecting left non-dominant side   1
I69.992-Facial weakness following unspecified cerebrovascular disease   1
I69.922-Dysarthria following unspecified cerebrovascular disease   1
I69.11-Cognitive deficits following nontraumatic intracerebral hemorrhage   1
I25.758-Atherosclerosis of native coronary artery of transplanted heart with other forms of angina pectoris   1
I22.8-Subsequent ST elevation (STEMI) myocardial infarction of other sites   1
I69.910-Attention and concentration deficit following unspecified cerebrovascular disease   1
410.61-POSTERIOR AMI-INIT EPISD   1
I63.513-Cerebral infarction due to unspecified occlusion or stenosis of bilateral middle cerebral arteries   1
I69.190-Apraxia following nontraumatic intracerebral hemorrhage   1
I63.543-Cerebral infarction due to unspecified occlusion or stenosis of bilateral cerebellar arteries   1
I69.192-Facial weakness following nontraumatic intracerebral hemorrhage   1
I69.021-Dysphasia following nontraumatic subarachnoid hemorrhage   1
I63.331-Cerebral infarction due to thrombosis of right posterior cerebral artery   1
I25.6-Silent myocardial ischemia   1
I63.341-Cerebral infarction due to thrombosis of right cerebellar artery   1
I63.19-Cerebral infarction due to embolism of other precerebral artery   1
I69.234-Monoplegia of upper limb following other nontraumatic intracranial hemorrhage affecting left non-dom.   1
I69.939-Monoplegia of upper limb following unspecified cerebrovascular disease affecting unspecified side   1
433.8-OCCL & STEN OF OTHER SPECIFIED PRECEREBRAL ARTERY   1
410.1-AMI ANTERIOR WALL NEC   1
I69.259-Hemiplegia and hemiparesis following other nontraumatic intracranial hemorrhage affecting unspecifie   1
I25.720-Atherosclerosis of autologous artery coronary artery bypass graft(s) with unstable angina pectoris   1
433.9-OCCL & STEN OF UNSPECIFIED PRECEREBRAL ARTERY   1
I63.6-Cerebral infarction due to cerebral venous thrombosis, nonpyogenic   1
440.31-ATHEROSCLEROSIS;AUTOLOGOUS VEIN BYPASS GFT;EXTREM.   1
I63.29-Cerebral infarction due to unspecified occlusion or stenosis of other precerebral arteries   1
I69.313-Psychomotor deficit following cerebral infarction   1
I69.10-Unspecified sequelae of nontraumatic intracerebral hemorrhage   1
414.06-OF NATIVE CORONARY ARTERY OF TRANSPLANTED HEART   1
I69.893-Ataxia following other cerebrovascular disease   1
I69.31-Cognitive deficits following cerebral infarction   1
434.1-CEREBRAL EMBOLISM   1
410.72-SUBENDO INFRC-LATR EPISD   1
I69.919-Unspecified symptoms and signs involving cognitive functions following unspecified cerebrovascular d   1
I69.322-Dysarthria following cerebral infarction   1

I69.920-Aphasia following unspecified cerebrovascular disease	1
434.0-CEREBRAL THROMBOSIS	1
I69.928-Other speech and language deficits following unspecified cerebrovascular disease	1
I69.331-Monoplegia of upper limb following cerebral infarction affecting right dominant side	1
I69.949-Monoplegia of lower limb following unspecified cerebrovascular disease affecting unspecified side	1
I63.011-Cerebral infarction due to thrombosis of right vertebral artery	1
I69.952-Hemiplegia and hemiparesis following unspecified cerebrovascular disease affecting left dominant sid	1
414.12-DISSECTION OF CORONARY ARTERY	1
I25.719-Atherosclerosis of autologous vein coronary artery bypass graft(s) with unspecified angina pectoris	1
I69.353-Hemiplegia and hemiparesis following cerebral infarction affecting right non-dominant side	1
I63.532-Cerebral infarction due to unspecified occlusion or stenosis of left posterior cerebral artery	1
I63.032-Cerebral infarction due to thrombosis of left carotid artery	1
I63.542-Cerebral infarction due to unspecified occlusion or stenosis of left cerebellar artery	1
I63.09-Cerebral infarction due to thrombosis of other precerebral artery	1
I25.739-Atherosclerosis of nonautologous biological coronary artery bypass graft(s) with unspecified angina	1
I63.441-Cerebral infarction due to embolism of right cerebellar artery	1
I63.81-Other cerebral infarction due to occlusion or stenosis of small artery	1
I63.443-Cerebral infarction due to embolism of bilateral cerebellar arteries	1
I25.798-Atherosclerosis of other coronary artery bypass graft(s) with other forms of angina pectoris	1
433.31-OCCL & STEN, MULT & BILAT ART W/CEREB INFARCT	1
I69.020-Aphasia following nontraumatic subarachnoid hemorrhage	1
I69.828-Other speech and language deficits following other cerebrovascular disease	1
I25.799-Atherosclerosis of other coronary artery bypass graft(s) with unspecified angina pectoris	1
I69.834-Monoplegia of upper limb following other cerebrovascular disease affecting left non-dominant side	1
I63.12-Cerebral infarction due to embolism of basilar artery	1
(blank)	
Grand Total	**16514**

EMR Primacy Can Threaten Data Access

A common belief is that the advent of the EMR is an unalloyed benefit to those interested in collecting and analyzing data to drive health care quality improvement and population health interventions. What is not fully realized is that, like any system or organization, the EMR has a narcissistic view of the world-bending information structure to support its commercial function even at the expense of the larger informatics ecosystem. In this section I will provide a few examples as a warning for my peers.

The Text Blob

In our system, we have had, in the past, data feeds from primary collection systems such as an echocardiographic collection system. Upon the rise of the hegemonic EMR system, new primary collection systems when implemented are funded to transfer information to the EMR, but the maintenance of other analytic consumers of that information are ignored in the vain hope that ultimately, one needs only to go to the EMR—the single source of truth—to obtain the information originating from the primary collection system.

However, the EMR sees its role as preserving data detail in the manner in which the individual clinician consumes it as a one-time visual perusal. The display of the atomic data of ejection fraction, aortic valve surface area, or cross-valve flow can be satisfied in the clinical physician perusal by the printing of that data by the primary system into a text blob, which is then manifested in the EMR as an image. But the original atomic nature is not retained, thereby functionally hiding this atomic data from cohort and outcome construction.

This process of blobization destroys structured data, delaying its availability until the advent of natural language processing. An institution wishing to maintain and extend analytic capability must explicitly consider this destructive proclivity and explicitly—with each upgrade of the source system—fund the maintenance of the atomic-level information for use in the enterprise data warehouse as a primary target of the analytic ecosystem. Leaving this responsibility to the EMR vendor is a guarantee of loss and mischief.

Forms and the Segregation of Data

Common constructs, such as depression scales, can appear in many intake forms in an EMR. Different departments, programs, or surveys may all be collecting information about depression using the same standardized scales and questions, but their intake forms are often created in blissful ignorance of other such efforts. This can cause identical information to be scattered in different variables and tables.

This thoughtless data-collection method functionally segregates information. Each new form hides data for another patient subgroup. While this allows an unsophisticated report writer to rapidly list or count the number of depressed patients in a specific department, it precludes the ease of analysis of the entire EMR population or reimagined subpopulations that cross departments.

A metadata strategy discipline ought to be a requirement of the EMR maintenance team to preserve a single variable in a single table for a common construct so that downstream analytic platforms can easily access that construct from one variable and table, rather than require a wild scramble foraging for hidden troves of depression information. This can be established in the original EMR, if it is sophisticated enough to support this commonality. If it is not, however, it must be enrolled in a common data target in an Enterprise Data warehouse with an accompanying clinical data dictionary. The time to do this is not the time of the query but at the time of enrollment of a new form or data-acquisition process—a task now "more honored in the breach than the observance" (*Hamlet* Act 1, scene iv).

"Before the Blind Do Not Put a Stumbling Block... and Thou Shalt Fear Thy G-d" (Leviticus 19:14)

n a recent study-design review session with a junior investigator, we discussed the issue of the power of the study. Power is the probability that, if the treatment effect you are trying to detect is of a certain size—say, a reduction of a negative outcome by 25%—your designed clinical trial has a reasonable chance (power=80%) to detect a significant difference. That is, if you performed the study as designed and the drug really works, you will see a statistically provable difference between the two treatments at least 80% of the time. Keep in mind this does not mean that the two treatments are 25% different in outcome, only that the outcomes are not the same.

This is a minimal requirement because you should not undertake a study unless both a negative and positive finding advance our knowledge. The negative result should add to our belief that there is no effect and we need not pursue the study of that therapy.

Power considerations therefore carry a heavy burden. Not only are the calculations permissive of the use of scarce resources in time, personnel, and attention, but also, if believed, they have the potential, in the case of a negative finding, to dissuade others from pursuing a therapy that might be of importance. As I have laid this out, power calculations are not just an annoying item to check off a list but carry a significant ethical burden.

In the course of the discussion, the investigator mentioned that he was advised by the pharmaceutical representative (an advocate for the study) that he should claim an effect of at least 25 percent because otherwise there would be inadequate power given the number of patients available.

We gently advised the investigator that, to put a fine point on it, the pharmaceutical representative had advised him to lie. Given the responsibility inherent in this calculation, he was advised to reconsider the effect size or study duration to achieve the power honestly.

Power discussions are arcane, and their considerations are hidden from the public view. The rabbis interpreted the biblical verse that leads this chapter as a warning that when you have knowledge that others lack, the other is metaphorically blind, and the metaphoric stumbling block is bad advice. Since only you and G-d know what is in your heart, you are proscribed from taking advantage of this situation to bend to your ends as there is a witness to your perfidious act.

A learning health system must own the hidden ethical decisions and sensitize its participants to their responsibility.

I Have Learned Many Things That Do Not Work

homas Edison was once taunted by a reporter who pointed out that he had failed thousands of times in his efforts to build an incandescent lightbulb. Edison is reported to have answered, "I have not failed; rather I have learned ten thousand things that do not work."

The purpose of a learning health system is to try new things and, in the process, to expect to fail. As long as each failure adds to the system's knowledge and changes its behavior, all is well.

I will describe broadly a few examples I have accumulated in discussion with peers in many institutions with slight exaggeration to make the point.

"But We Needed the N!" Pediatric Asthma Intervention in the ED

An intervention was planned to introduce intensive education and coordination for children who present with asthma to the emergency room. The initial project restricted the patients to those of a certain age with a history of significant asthma, inclusive of multiple ED or inpatient stays. Staffing was for a single nurse full time equivalent (FTE) waiting in the emergency department nine to five, five days a week to identify and intervene.

You may already begin to see the folly of the design and the impossible pressure placed upon the participants leading to corruption in project execution. As you might imagine, asthma does not restrict itself to a nine-to-five time window. This is especially true in children who need to be brought in by their caregivers. The caregivers' job constraints might force the visit to occur after normal work hours, making later hours more appropriate.

What was clearly missing was a check of the actual history of the emergency department asthma presentation times in the past to guide time selection. Also, a single staff member has sick, vacation, and family leave time, so by the time you are finished, you are looking at about six weeks of noncoverage each year for any single employee.

What happened next? The implementers recognized that they were not accruing patients fast enough, so they altered the inclusion requirement. Now, they no longer required asthmatics with significant emergency department or hospitalization history. They included the less sick. Thus, they included children with less opportunity for any intervention to manifest an effect. While getting the N they wanted, they functionally changed the study question and compromised the power of their efforts to manifest any meaningful result.

"Let's Put Some PharmDs in a Clinic!"

Historically, failure of adherence to medication is a major impediment to effective control of pharmaceutically remediable risk factors like high blood pressure or elevated cholesterol. In many of these situations, it is believed that what might be effective is the placement of a medication educator or pharmacy PhD in the clinic. After the educators were put into place for a period of time, the clinic wanted to look at the effect of this intervention on blood pressure control.

Of course, because it was not preplanned properly for evaluation, there was no control group. Meaningfulness of pre- and postdesigns suffered from regression to the mean. Propensity matching suffered from the missing variable problem.

Ignoring this control group problem and further accepting, for the sake of argument, that placing a pharmacy educator in a clinic during work hours is a reasonable intervention, this intervention suffers from a serious deficiency—a deficiency that is all too common.

While the analysis of the intervention appropriately considered the blood pressure months after the change in staffing, there was no intermediate process measure for repeat blood pressure checks before the end of the evaluation period. There was no surveillance of the process of care to identify those who were not actively engaged. This is an implementation error and should have been part of the design as such surveillance would have afforded the opportunity for outreach, which could have been part of the implementation strategy. It would potentially have provided early warning that the educator intervention was not an adequate engagement modifier and was failing early to achieve the adherence required for success.

Put in a Navigator, but Don't Give Her the Tools

In an effort to prevent unnecessary hospital admissions, health systems have placed navigators in the emergency room to meet defined patients, potentially preventing their admission by arranging for alternatives. The location in the emergency room is an interesting choice and, in a sense, a last-ditch effort. As was discussed in the chapter "Observed vs. True Cost Savings: Why Health Systems Do Not Evolve," it is preferable to intervene even earlier. This is particularly true in patients whose symptoms have been detected at home prior to the emergency room presentation.

Navigator effectiveness is dependent upon a number of capabilities. First, the navigator must be able to rapidly identify the patient once he presents to the emergency department either through an active referral by staff or by some automated method that identifies those patients whose profile indicates an enhanced clinical need.

Second, the nurse navigator must have specific resources for specific problems whose resolution might prevent admission. If, for example, a rapid specialist appointment might preclude the admission, then the ability to guarantee that appointment first thing the next day is such a capability. If the patient needs a specific social support, then having access, not only to a social worker but to specific service capabilities to be delivered immediately to the home—be it a visiting nurse, medication delivery, social support, an aid, or a visiting physician—then makes it possible for the navigator to activate these options. In turn, this supports the possibility of admission prevention.

The scenarios must be planned for with specific actionable resources that can be brought to bear in real time. Merely putting a nurse in the emergency room to send an electronic request for a consult that will be assessed the next day at some time for an indeterminate date of resolution is a fake solution.

If, in fact, these options are not enabled, or that if initially enabled, but over time dissipate, then the nurse navigator program continues in the sense that there is a physical body present, but her activities are redirected to needs other than the primary focus. Establishing surveillance of her interventions and their outcomes is therefore not so much a surveillance of the performance of the individual nurse navigator as an employee. Rather it is a surveillance of the integrity of the health system in providing admission prophylaxis in the full sense of assessing the nurse navigator and supportive structure.

If the Only Tool You Have is a Hammer, the Whole World Looks Like a Nail

I asked a colleague who works in the grant infrastructure of the federal government why the language of the long-term surveillance of disease was always focused on the doctor and his office relationship with the patient. Follow-up of cancer care for appropriate subsequent screening tests or prophylaxis on the order of years requires a system that might be exogenous of the originating physician and her office. You can imagine that at year five post treatment, that physician might no longer be in the office, and the patient may no longer be interacting with the original information system. Thus, trying to reach that physician or that patient for patient follow-up care five years later through the original EMR would be an exercise in futility.

I suggested that grant funding for the purpose of long-term follow-up care should create a registration system outside the original EMR (exogenous), and that system should be charged with maintaining a relationship with the patient, knowing where he is and how to reach him. Registration in such an exogenous surveillance system would be voluntary but would offer the patient the benefit of being informed about new protocols and the need for timely follow-up care.

The response I was given was telling. "As funders, we cannot modify the infrastructure. We live in the world as it is, so we must fund projects that utilize the existing infrastructure, even if in some sense, it is inadequately designed for the required purpose." Consider what this means: a universe of federal funding continues to fund false premises because of the convenience in conformity with the limitations of the present. There is no reprieve visible on the horizon.

If I Am a Success, Why Should I Change?

The world adapts to its own reality. It is the perfect world for the present configuration of things. But what if that configuration is wrong? We confuse our present success with our own skill and insight, a point made clear by the quip, "He was born on third base and thinks he hit a triple."

Success does not mean that you should continue what you are doing. You may be successful despite yourself and certainly may not have maximally learned from the reality around you.

CONCLUSION

O nce the health system develops a consciousness and assumes responsibility for outcomes on even the most primitive level, it is, by nature of this responsibility, required to assume management of some of the assets—people and resources.

As a first step, episodic acute care such as the episode of elective hip replacement naturally falls under sway. The preoperative evaluation, intraoperative equipment and materials, postoperative physical therapy, or rehabilitation is bundled into a system deliverable with cost accountability transferred to the big dog receiver of dollars: the hospital. The interval of care is given a fixed payment, and any readmission or unexpected complication is the responsibility of the hospital. This model works well when there is a defined aliquot of a high-profit deliverable over a limited time duration. Simple economic incentives and market negotiation with a powerful aware and active payor can drive down the costs and increase episode efficiency. However, when the episodes of care are more long lived—with longitudinal health care and a less-intense payment—the machinery needed to evolve to support efficient care needs fine-tuned management with intense learning and then decision making as to what efforts to undertake at what nonreimbursable cost. This does not arise spontaneously.

The spontaneous hip fracture case makes this point really clear. A patient fractures her hip while playing tennis on a visit to Florida. The hip is pinned in Florida with an aliquot of payment to the hospital and physicians there. Upon returning to New Jersey, the patient seeks postoperative and longitudinal care for her fracture. What does she discover? No orthopedist is interested in assuming her care, despite multiple phone calls. A new, nationally recognized specialty group that recently moved into her geographic area was unable or unwilling after multiple searches to find a member of its staff to take on this task. Why? Because the big money for the episode had already been made. The follow-up care is performed at a loss that is sustained only because it enables the bucks of the initial procedure. When I discussed this case with the patient, the conversation focused on whether the stitches should be removed by her internist or a physician assistant and not what this clinical event meant for follow-up intervention given her evident osteoporosis manifesting in a fracture. Besides the physical therapy, what is to be done about bone-preservation therapy alendronate and zoledronic acid? When should these medications be started? Now or in a few weeks? Where is the protocol, the collaborative expertise of the surgeon, internist, and endocrinologist, either by an established joint algorithm or the coordinated consultation to assume care and advise?

Economics does not create in and of itself the needed organized, responsible, and learning health care system. The invisible-hand economics currently in play creates a predatory system that builds service delivery systems to feast on the high-yielding procedures, eschewing necessary nonremunerative ones unless they are bundled by force of convention or contract.

As systems become aware and begin to assume responsibility, the extent of that responsibility is identified through articulated questions. Questions can only be articulated if three elements are present: the desire to learn, the desire to act, and the ability to access and organize data to support the learning. The more enabled a system is to ask questions, the more it reveals its inadequacies. This is a tough place for management to live. Management's blissful ignorance, whether by accident or by design, especially when it can hide in the shared mediocrity of other health care systems, allows it to claim adequacy and success based on the observables of size and public image.

Management can make subtle decisions to protect itself from awareness. It can choose not to develop a repository of data or an analytic tool that allows for the creation of cohorts and outcome evaluation without the intercession of an analytic priesthood. It can fail to reinforce a systematic demand for self-reflection and the implementation of interventions. It can penalize those who discover problems and reward those who do not bring new problems, especially those with cost up the command chain for awareness. There can be either an implicit or explicit message from higher management that it is happy when subordinates so well manage their domain that no issues need to reach upper management.

This is a dishonest standard as the infrastructure and process engineering necessary to address some of the issues discussed in this book are only resolvable with shared resources funded by an aware senior management team amortizing engineered resource cost across multiple departments and multiple initiatives to achieve cost effectiveness. Not all issues deserve equal attention. No organization has the budget to solve all problems, but the proper balance of surfacing, engaging, considering, and prioritizing is a critical responsibility of management.

In this book, I have provided examples of the sort of analyses that are possible when you have the proper data collection, a tool for cohort analysis and outcomes, and the will to ask.

In no way am I claiming that we have solved the LHS management problem, for it is both dynamic and new without clear historical guidance, but we have begun to articulate some of these questions with the help of Clinical Looking Glass, and I hope that by sharing some elements of our early journey, we will help other systems decide what they want to know and what they are prepared to do as they evolve into a learning health system that learns, decides, and acts.

ACKNOWLEDGMENTS

would like to acknowledge important conversations and shared projects over the years with Devin Thompson, David Esses, Chinazo Cunningham, Joanna Starrels, John Bianco

David Esses, Bryan W. Lewis, Lindsay Stahl, Stephen Kulovits, Ladan Golestaneh, Urvashi Patel, Michael Baker, Donna Lusardi, Scott Monrad, and Daniel Labovitz.

While my debt to those acknowledged for their insight and suggestions is deep, any error of analysis or presentation is mine alone.

BIBLIOGRAPHY

1. Smith MD, Institute of Medicine (U.S.). Committee on the Learning Health Care System in America. *Best care at lower cost : the path to continuously learning health care in America.* Washington, D.C.: National Academies Press; 2013.

2. Bellin E, Fletcher DD, Geberer N, Islam S, Srivastava N. Democratizing information creation from health care data for quality improvement, research, and education—the Montefiore Medical Center experience. *Academic Medicine.* 2010;85(8):1362-1368.

3. Bellin E. *How to ask and answer questions using electronic medical record data.* South Carolina: Create Space; 2017.

4. Bellin E. *Riddles in Accountable Healthcare: A primer to develop analytic intuition for medical homes and population health.* South Carolina: Create Space; 2015.

5. Katsuyama j. Doctor tells patient he doesn't have long to live through hospital robot's video screen. KTVU.com. http://www.fox5ny.com/news/doctor-tells-patient-he-doesn-t-have-long-to-live-through-hospital-robot-s-video-screen. Published 2019. AccessedMay 5, 2019.

6. Felsen UR, Bellin EY, Cunningham CO, Zingman BS. Unknown HIV Status in the Emergency Department: Implications for Expanded Testing Strategies. *J Int Assoc Provid AIDS Care.* 2015.

7. Bellin E, Fletcher DD, Geberer N, Islam S, Srivastava N. Democratizing information creation from health care data for quality improvement, research, and education-the Montefiore Medical Center Experience. *Acad Med.* 2010;85(8):1362-1368.

8. Banegas JR, Ruilope LM, de la Sierra A, et al. Relationship between Clinic and Ambulatory Blood-Pressure Measurements and Mortality. *N Engl J Med.* 2018;378(16):1509-1520.

9.   Frieden TR. SHATTUCK LECTURE: The Future of Public Health. *N Engl J Med.* 2015;373(18):1748-1754.

10.   Farley TA, Dalal MA, Mostashari F, Frieden TR. Deaths preventable in the U.S. by improvements in use of clinical preventive services. *Am J Prev Med.* 2010;38(6):600-609.

11.   Chobanian AV. Shattuck Lecture. The hypertension paradox--more uncontrolled disease despite improved therapy. *N Engl J Med.* 2009;361(9):878-887.

12.   Diez Roux AV, Merkin SS, Arnett D, et al. Neighborhood of residence and incidence of coronary heart disease. *N Engl J Med.* 2001;345(2):99-106.

13.   Powers BJ, Olsen MK, Smith VA, Woolson RF, Bosworth HB, Oddone EZ. Measuring blood pressure for decision making and quality reporting: where and how many measures? *Ann Intern Med.* 2011;154(12):781-788, W-289-790.

14.   Williams B, Lindholm LH, Sever P. Systolic pressure is all that matters. *Lancet.* 2008;371(9631):2219-2221.

15.   Myers MG. A proposed algorithm for diagnosing hypertension using automated office blood pressure measurement. *J Hypertens.* 2010;28(4):703-708.

16.   Pickering TG, Shimbo D, Haas D. Ambulatory blood-pressure monitoring. *N Engl J Med.* 2006;354(22):2368-2374.

17.   Sega R, Facchetti R, Bombelli M, et al. Prognostic value of ambulatory and home blood pressures compared with office blood pressure in the general population: follow-up results from the Pressioni Arteriose Monitorate e Loro Associazioni (PAMELA) study. *Circulation.* 2005;111(14):1777-1783.

18.   Kikuya M, Ohkubo T, Asayama K, et al. Ambulatory blood pressure and 10-year risk of cardiovascular and noncardiovascular mortality: the Ohasama study. *Hypertension.* 2005;45(2):240-245.

19.   Dolan E, Stanton A, Thijs L, et al. Superiority of ambulatory over clinic blood pressure measurement in predicting mortality: the Dublin outcome study. *Hypertension.* 2005;46(1):156-161.

20.   Clement DL, De Buyzere ML, De Bacquer DA, et al. Prognostic value of ambulatory blood-pressure recordings in patients with treated hypertension. *N Engl J Med.* 2003;348(24):2407-2415.

21.   Staessen JA, Thijs L, Fagard R, et al. Predicting cardiovascular risk using conventional vs ambulatory blood pressure in older patients with systolic hypertension. Systolic Hypertension in Europe Trial Investigators. *JAMA.* 1999;282(6):539-546.

22.   James PA, Oparil S, Carter BL, et al. 2014 evidence-based guideline for the management of high blood pressure in adults: report from the panel members appointed to the Eighth Joint National Committee (JNC 8). *JAMA.* 2014;311(5):507-520.

23.   Cohen P, Cohen J. The clinician's illusion. *Arch Gen Psychiatry.* 1984;41(12):1178-1182.

24.   Kaplan EL, Meier,P. Nonparametric estimation from incomplete observations. *J Amer Statist Assoc.*53(282):457-481.

25.   Efron B, Tibshirani R. *An introduction to the bootstrap.* New York: Chapman & Hall; 1993.

26.   Verberk WJ, Kroon AA, Lenders JW, et al. Self-measurement of blood pressure at home reduces the need for antihypertensive drugs: a randomized, controlled trial. *Hypertension.* 2007;50(6):1019-1025.

27.   Centers for Disease C, Prevention. Vital signs: avoidable deaths from heart disease, stroke, and hypertensive disease - United States, 2001-2010. *MMWR Morb Mortal Wkly Rep.* 2013;62(35):721-727.

28. Box GEP, Hunter,J.S,Hunter,W.G. *Statistics for Experimenters.* 2nd ed: John Wiley & Sons; 2005.

29. Turner BJ, Hollenbeak CS, Weiner M, Ten Have T, Tang SS. Effect of unrelated comorbid conditions on hypertension management. *Ann Intern Med.* 2008;148(8):578-586.

30. Phillips LS, Twombly JG. It's time to overcome clinical inertia. *Ann Intern Med.* 2008;148(10):783-785.

31. Clemens SL. *The prince and the pauper.* Chicago, The John C. Winston company,1937.

32. Codman EA. *A study in hospital efficiency : as demonstrated by the case report of the first five years of a private hospital.* Oakbrook Terrace, IL: Joint Commission on Accreditation of Healthcare Organizations; 1996.

33. Saywell RM, Jr., Champion VL, Skinner CS, Menon U, Daggy J. A cost-effectiveness comparison of three tailored interventions to increase mammography screening. *J Womens Health (Larchmt).* 2004;13(8):909-918.

34. Davis NA, Nash E, Bailey C, Lewis MJ, Rimer BK, Koplan JP. Evaluation of three methods for improving mammography rates in a managed care plan. *Am J Prev Med.* 1997;13(4):298-302.

35. Thaler RH, Sunstein CR. *Nudge : improving decisions about health, wealth, and happiness.* Rev. and expanded ed. New York: Penguin Books; 2009.

36. Wheeler DJ, Chambers DS. *Understanding statistical process control.* 3rd ed. Knoxville, Tenn.: SPC Press; 2010.

37. Grant EL, Leavenworth RS. *Statistical quality control.* 7th ed. New York: McGraw-Hill Co. Inc.; 1996.

38. Qiu P. *Introduction to Statistical Process Control.* New York: CRC Press; 2014.

39.   Carey RG, Lloyd RC. *Quality with confidence in healthcare : a practical guide to quality improvement in healthcare.* Chicago, IL: SPSS; 1997.

40.   Ody C, Msall L, Dafny LS, Grabowski DC, Cutler DM. Decreases In Readmissions Credited To Medicare's Program To Reduce Hospital Readmissions Have Been Overstated. *Health affairs.* 2019;38(1):36-43.

41.   Goldratt EM, Cox J, Goldratt EM. *The goal : a process of ongoing improvement.* Fourth revised edition, 30th anniversary edition. ed.

42.   Deming WE. *Out of the crisis.* Reissue. ed. Cambridge, Massachsetts: The MIT Press; 2018.

43.   Quan H, Sundararajan V, Halfon P, et al. Coding algorithms for defining comorbidities in ICD-9-CM and ICD-10 administrative data. *Medical care.* 2005;43(11):1130-1139.

44.   Charlson ME, Pompei P, Ales KL, MacKenzie CR. A new method of classifying prognostic comorbidity in longitudinal studies: development and validation. *Journal of chronic diseases.* 1987;40(5):373-383.

45.   Tremblay D, Arnsten JH, Southern WN. A Simple and Powerful Risk-Adjustment Tool for 30-day Mortality Among Inpatients. *Qual Manag Health Care.* 2016;25(3):123-128.

46.   Quan H, Li B, Couris CM, et al. Updating and validating the Charlson comorbidity index and score for risk adjustment in hospital discharge abstracts using data from 6 countries. *Am J Epidemiol.* 2011;173(6):676-682.

47.   James GW, Daniela,;Hastie,Trevor; Tibshirani, Robert. *An Introduction to Statistical Learning: with Applications in R.* New York: Springer; 2013.

48.   Segal M, Pedersen AL, Freeman K, Fast A. Medicare's new restrictions on rehabilitation admissions: impact on the elderly. *Am J Phys Med Rehabil.* 2008;87(11):872-882.

49.   Guy GP, Jr., Zhang K, Schieber LZ, Young R, Dowell D. County-Level Opioid Prescribing in the United States, 2015 and 2017. *JAMA Intern Med.* 2019.

50.   Schieber LZ, Guy GP, Jr., Seth P, et al. Trends and Patterns of Geographic Variation in Opioid Prescribing Practices by State, United States, 2006-2017. *JAMA Netw Open.* 2019;2(3):e190665.

51.   Health NYSDo. I-Stop/PMP - Internet System for Tracking Over-Prescribing-Prescription Monitoring Program. https://www.health.ny.gov/professionals/narcotic/prescription_monitoring/. Published 2019. Accessed2019.

52.   Golestaneh L, Alvarez PJ, Reaven NL, et al. All-cause costs increase exponentially with increased chronic kidney disease stage. *Am J Manag Care.* 2017;23(10 Suppl):S163-S172.

53.   Heerspink HJL, Parving HH, Andress DL, et al. Atrasentan and renal events in patients with type 2 diabetes and chronic kidney disease (SONAR): a double-blind, randomised, placebo-controlled trial. *Lancet.* 2019.

54.   McFarland LV, Mulligan ME, Kwok RY, Stamm WE. Nosocomial acquisition of Clostridium difficile infection. *N Engl J Med.* 1989;320(4):204-210.

55.   Bartlett JG, Chang TW, Gurwith M, Gorbach SL, Onderdonk AB. Antibiotic-associated pseudomembranous colitis due to toxin-producing clostridia. *N Engl J Med.* 1978;298(10):531-534.

56.   Nolan NP, Kelly CP, Humphreys JF, et al. An epidemic of pseudomembranous colitis: importance of person to person spread. *Gut.* 1987;28(11):1467-1473.

57.   Pierce PF, Jr., Wilson R, Silva J, Jr., et al. Antibiotic-associated pseudomembranous colitis: an epidemiologic investigation of a cluster of cases. *The Journal of infectious diseases.* 1982;145(2):269-274.

58.   Gabriel L, Beriot-Mathiot A. Hospitalization stay and costs attributable to Clostridium difficile infection: a critical review. *J Hosp Infect.* 2014;88(1):12-21.

59.   Johnson S, Gerding DN, Olson MM, et al. Prospective, controlled study of vinyl glove use to interrupt Clostridium difficile nosocomial transmission. *Am J Med.* 1990;88(2):137-140.

60.   Edmonds SL, Zapka C, Kasper D, et al. Effectiveness of hand hygiene for removal of Clostridium difficile spores from hands. *Infection control and hospital epidemiology : the official journal of the Society of Hospital Epidemiologists of America.* 2013;34(3):302-305.

61.   Kelly CP, LaMont JT. Clostridium difficile--more difficult than ever. *N Engl J Med.* 2008;359(18):1932-1940.

62.   Svenungsson B, Burman LG, Jalakas-Pornull K, Lagergren A, Struwe J, Akerlund T. Epidemiology and molecular characterization of Clostridium difficile strains from patients with diarrhea: low disease incidence and evidence of limited cross-infection in a Swedish teaching hospital. *Journal of clinical microbiology.* 2003;41(9):4031-4037.

63.   Wullt M, Laurell MH. Low prevalence of nosocomial Clostridium difficile transmission, as determined by comparison of arbitrarily primed PCR and epidemiological data. *J Hosp Infect.* 1999;43(4):265-273.

64.   Walker AS, Eyre DW, Wyllie DH, et al. Characterisation of Clostridium difficile hospital ward-based transmission using extensive epidemiological data and molecular typing. *PLoS medicine.* 2012;9(2):e1001172.

65.   Hamel M, Zoutman D, O'Callaghan C. Exposure to hospital roommates as a risk factor for health care-associated infection. *Am J Infect Control.* 2010;38(3):173-181.

66.   Dubberke ER, Reske KA, Olsen MA, et al. Evaluation of Clostridium difficile-associated disease pressure as a risk factor for C difficile-associated disease. *Arch Intern Med.* 2007;167(10):1092-1097.

67.   Yu B, Wang Zo. Estimating relative risks for common outcome using PROC NLP. *Computer Methods and Programs in Biomedicine.* 2008;90:7.

68.   *est.rr Relative Risk. The R project for statistical computing* [computer program]. 2009.

69.   Hosmer DW, Lemeshow S, Sturdivant RX. *Applied Logistic Regression*. Hoboken, N.J.: John Wiley & Sons, Inc.; 2013.

70.   Lemeshow S, Hosmer DW. The use of goodness-of-fit statistics in the development of logistic regression models. *American Journal of Epidemiology*. 1982;115:92-106.

71.   Hosmer DW, Lemeshow S. A goodness-of-fit test for the multiple logistic regression model. *Communications in Statistics*. 1980;A10:1043-1069.

72.   Austin PC. Absolute risk reductions, relative risks, relative risk reductions, and numbers needed to treat can be obtained from a logistic regression model. *Journal of clinical epidemiology*. 2010;63(1):2-6.

73.   Cook RJ, Sackett DL. The number needed to treat: a clinically useful measure of treatment effect. *Bmj*. 1995;310(6977):452-454.

74.   Curry SR, Muto CA, Schlackman JL, et al. Use of multilocus variable number of tandem repeats analysis genotyping to determine the role of asymptomatic carriers in Clostridium difficile transmission. *Clin Infect Dis*. 2013;57(8):1094-1102.

75.   McDonald LC, Coignard B, Dubberke E, et al. Recommendations for surveillance of Clostridium difficile-associated disease. *Infection control and hospital epidemiology : the official journal of the Society of Hospital Epidemiologists of America*. 2007;28(2):140-145.

76.   Carter AA, Gomes T, Camacho X, Juurlink DN, Shah BR, Mamdani MM. Risk of incident diabetes among patients treated with statins: population based study. *Bmj*. 2013;346:f2610.

77.   Culver AL, Ockene IS, Ma Y. Statin use and risk of diabetes-reply. *Arch Intern Med*. 2012;172(11):896-897.

78. Ma Y, Culver A, Rossouw J, et al. Statin therapy and the risk for diabetes among adult women: do the benefits outweigh the risk? *Therapeutic advances in cardiovascular disease.* 2013;7(1):41-44.

79. Preiss D, Seshasai SR, Welsh P, et al. Risk of incident diabetes with intensive-dose compared with moderate-dose statin therapy: a meta-analysis. *JAMA.* 2011;305(24):2556-2564.

80. Sattar N, Preiss D, Murray HM, et al. Statins and risk of incident diabetes: a collaborative meta-analysis of randomised statin trials. *Lancet.* 2010;375(9716):735-742.

81. Culver AL, Ockene IS, Balasubramanian R, et al. Statin use and risk of diabetes mellitus in postmenopausal women in the Women's Health Initiative. *Arch Intern Med.* 2012;172(2):144-152.

82. Sever PS, Dahlof B, Poulter NR, et al. Prevention of coronary and stroke events with atorvastatin in hypertensive patients who have average or lower-than-average cholesterol concentrations, in the Anglo-Scandinavian Cardiac Outcomes Trial--Lipid Lowering Arm (ASCOT-LLA): a multicentre randomised controlled trial. *Lancet.* 2003;361(9364):1149-1158.

83. Colhoun HM, Betteridge DJ, Durrington PN, et al. Primary prevention of cardiovascular disease with atorvastatin in type 2 diabetes in the Collaborative Atorvastatin Diabetes Study (CARDS): multicentre randomised placebo-controlled trial. *Lancet.* 2004;364(9435):685-696.

84. Cox AJ, Hsu FC, Freedman BI, et al. Contributors to Mortality in High-Risk Diabetic Patients in the Diabetes Heart Study. *Diabetes care.* 2014.

85. Iacus SM, King, G, and Porro, G. Multivariate Matching Methods that are Monotonic Imbalance Bounding. *Journal of the American Statistical Association.* 2011;106(106):345-361.

86. Sekhon J. Genetic Optimization Using Derivatives: The rgenoud package for R. *Journal of Statistical Software.* 2011;42(11):1-26.

87. Lin M, Lucas HC, Shmueli G. Research Commentary—Too Big to Fail: Large Samples and the p-Value Problem. *Information Systems Research.* 2013;24(4):906-917.

88. Balakrishnan N, Rao C. Advances in Survival Analysis. In: Rao C, ed. *Handbook of Statistics 23: Advances in Survival Analysis.* Vol 23. New York: Elsevier; 2004:795.

89. Bellin E, Fletcher DD, Geberer N, Islam S, Srivastava N. Democratizing information creation from health care data for quality improvement, research, and education-the Montefiore Medical Center Experience. *AcadMed.* 2010;85(8):1362-1368.

90. Action to Control Cardiovascular Risk in Diabetes Study G, Gerstein HC, Miller ME, et al. Effects of intensive glucose lowering in type 2 diabetes. *N Engl J Med.* 2008;358(24):2545-2559.

91. Group AS, Gerstein HC, Miller ME, et al. Long-term effects of intensive glucose lowering on cardiovascular outcomes. *N Engl J Med.* 2011;364(9):818-828.

92. Hersh W. Beyond prediction: Data analytics/ Data Science / Big Data must demonstrate value. http://informaticsprofessor.blogspot.com/2014/08/beyond-prediction-data-analyticsdata.html. Published 2014. Accessed 9/7/2014, 2014.

93. Arnold T, Kane M, Lewis BW. *A computational approach to statistical learning.* Boca Raton: Taylor & Francis, CRC Press; 2019.

94. James G, Witten D, Hastie T, Tibshirani R. An Introduction to Statistical Learning with Applications in R. In: *Springer Texts in Statistics,.*

95. Hastie T, Tibshirani R, Friedman J. The Elements of Statistical Learning Data Mining, Inference, and Prediction. In: *Springer Series in Statistics,.* 2nd ed.

96. van der Laan MJ, Rose S. Targeted Learning in Data Science Causal Inference for Complex Longitudinal Studies. In: *Springer Series in Statistics,.*

97. van der Laan MJ, Rose S. Targeted Learning Causal Inference for Observational and Experimental Data. In: *Springer Series in Statistics,.*

98.   Efron B, Hastie T. *Computer age statistical inference : algorithms, evidence, and data science.* New York, NY: Cambridge University Press; 2016.

99.   Goodfellow I, Bengio Y, Courville A. *Deep learning.* Cambridge, Massachusetts: The MIT Press; 2016.

100. Marsland S. *Machine learning : an algorithmic perspective.* Second edition. ed. Boca Raton: CRC Press; 2015.

101. Steyerberg EW, Vergouwe Y. Towards better clinical prediction models: seven steps for development and an ABCD for validation. *Eur Heart J.* 2014;35(29):1925-1931.

102. Escobar GJ, Greene JD, Scheirer P, Gardner MN, Draper D, Kipnis P. Risk-adjusting hospital inpatient mortality using automated inpatient, outpatient, and laboratory databases. *Medical care.* 2008;46(3):232-239.

103. Rajkomar A, Oren E, Chen K, et al. Scalable and accurate deep learning with electronic health records. *npj Digital Medicine.* 2018;1(1):18.

104. Dziadzko MA, Novotny PJ, Sloan J, et al. Multicenter derivation and validation of an early warning score for acute respiratory failure or death in the hospital. *Critical Care.* 2018;22(1):286.

105. Lam MB, Figueroa JF, Feyman Y, Reimold KE, Orav EJ, Jha AK. Association between patient outcomes and accreditation in US hospitals: observational study. *Bmj.* 2018;363:k4011.

106. Pandey A, Golwala H, Hall HM, et al. Association of US Centers for Medicare and Medicaid Services Hospital 30-Day Risk-Standardized Readmission Metric With Care Quality and Outcomes After Acute Myocardial Infarction: Findings From the National Cardiovascular Data Registry/Acute Coronary Treatment and Intervention Outcomes Network Registry-Get With the Guidelines. *JAMA Cardiol.* 2017;2(7):723-731.

107. Pandey A, Golwala H, Xu H, et al. Association of 30-Day Readmission Metric for Heart Failure Under the Hospital Readmissions Reduction Program With Quality of Care and Outcomes. *JACC Heart Fail.* 2016;4(12):935-946.

108. Zulman DM, Pal Chee C, Ezeji-Okoye SC, et al. Effect of an Intensive Outpatient Program to Augment Primary Care for High-Need Veterans Affairs Patients: A Randomized Clinical Trial. *JAMA Intern Med.* 2017;177(2):166-175.

109. Katz MH. Trust but Verify (Ideally With a Randomized Clinical Trial). *JAMA Intern Med.* 2017;177(2):162-163.

110. Golestaneh L. Decreasing hospitalizations in patients on hemodialysis: Time for a paradigm shift. *Semin Dial.* 2018;31(3):278-288.

111. Golestaneh L, Bellin E, Southern W, Melamed ML. Discharge service as a determinant of 30-day readmission in a cohort of maintenance hemodialysis patients: a retrospective cohort study. *BMC Nephrol.* 2017;18(1):352.

112. R [computer program]. Version 3.4.2: cran; 2017.

113. Smith GC, Pell JP. Parachute use to prevent death and major trauma related to gravitational challenge: systematic review of randomised controlled trials. *Bmj.* 2003;327(7429):1459-1461.

114. Chaudhry SI, Mattera JA, Curtis JP, et al. Telemonitoring in patients with heart failure. *N Engl J Med.* 2010;363(24):2301-2309.

115. Bogle JC. *Common sense on mutual funds : new imperatives for the intelligent investor.* New York: John Wiley; 1999.

116. Bellin E, Dubler NN. The quality improvement-research divide and the need for external oversight. *AmJPublic Health.* 2001;91(9):1512-1517.

117. Wilson FP, Parikh CR. Translational Methods in Nephrology: Individual Treatment Effect Modeling. *J Am Soc Nephrol.* 2018;29(11):2615-2618.

118. Group SR, Wright JT, Jr., Williamson JD, et al. A Randomized Trial of Intensive versus Standard Blood-Pressure Control. *N Engl J Med.* 2015;373(22):2103-2116.

119. Cholesterol Treatment Trialists C, Mihaylova B, Emberson J, et al. The effects of lowering LDL cholesterol with statin therapy in people at low risk of vascular disease: meta-analysis of individual data from 27 randomised trials. *Lancet.* 2012;380(9841):581-590.

120. Silverman MG, Ference BA, Im K, et al. Association Between Lowering LDL-C and Cardiovascular Risk Reduction Among Different Therapeutic Interventions: A Systematic Review and Meta-analysis. *JAMA.* 2016;316(12):1289-1297.

121. Cholesterol Treatment Trialists C, Baigent C, Blackwell L, et al. Efficacy and safety of more intensive lowering of LDL cholesterol: a meta-analysis of data from 170,000 participants in 26 randomised trials. *Lancet.* 2010;376(9753):1670-1681.

122. Lloyd-Jones DM, Braun LT, Ndumele CE, et al. Use of Risk Assessment Tools to Guide Decision-Making in the Primary Prevention of Atherosclerotic Cardiovascular Disease: A Special Report From the American Heart Association and American College of Cardiology. *J Am Coll Cardiol.* 2018.

123. Hayward RA, Hofer TP, Vijan S. Narrative review: lack of evidence for recommended low-density lipoprotein treatment targets: a solvable problem. *Ann Intern Med.* 2006;145(7):520-530.

124. Kane SP. Pooled Cohort Risk Assessment Equations. ClinicCalc, LLC. Evidence-based clinical decision support tools and calculators for medical professionals Web site. https://clincalc.com/Cardiology/ASCVD/PooledCohort.aspx. Published 2019. Accessed2019.

125. Goff DC, Jr., Lloyd-Jones DM, Bennett G, et al. 2013 ACC/AHA guideline on the assessment of cardiovascular risk: a report of the American College of Cardiology/American Heart Association Task Force on Practice Guidelines. *J Am Coll Cardiol.* 2014;63(25 Pt B):2935-2959.

www.ingramcontent.com/pod-product-compliance
Lightning Source LLC
Chambersburg PA
CBHW060828170526
45158CB00001B/115